HANNAH AN
WITH SCOTT BALDYGA

Living the
INVISIBLE
DISABILITY
COPING WITH POST CONCUSSION SYNDROME
TRAUMATIC BRAIN INJURY & DEPRESSION

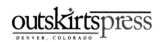

outskirtspress

DENVER, COLORADO

FOREWORD

I entered medical school at 19 and soon realized neurology was in some ways the most interesting of all clinical specialties. What a remarkable organ the brain is! It has the power to create a mind, with emotions, memories, desires, aversions, symbolism and seman- tics—all the things for which minds are noted. In fact, we each have two brains, corresponding to the left and right hemispheres of our brains, and to a large extent we have two minds, which emerge when the left and right hemispheres are separated by surgery, trauma, or agenesis of the corpus callosum (a structure that normally joins the hemispheres together).

How is a mind generated by brain activity? This question has never been answered in a way that would satisfy most of us, and the artificial creation of a mind remains far beyond the reach of technol- ogy today. We must admit we don't really know. In the 4th century BC, Aristotle proclaimed that the heart was the seat of intelligence, whereas the brain was principally responsible for cooling the blood. And even to the present day, popular banter suggests that the "heart- as-seat-of-emotions" idea is not quite dead. Our modern view that brains create minds arose and endured because physical injuries to brains reproducibly disrupt mental function. We even know what kind of mental abnormality to expect when one part of the brain is damaged as opposed to another. The development of imaging tech- nologies, some of which are mentioned in this book, has recently enhanced our understanding of which parts of the brain do what. Yet much remains unclear, and damage to the brain, subtle or even undetectable by our most sensitive instrumentation, can have genuine consequences for the mind. Some of these consequences may be reversible; some possibly not. Unique among organs, the brain remembers its past, and is influenced by the traumas it has borne, even when no anatomic trace of pathology remains.

Hannah Andrusky, whom I knew very well before, during, and since her ordeal, describes what a post-concussive injury was like for her. Objectively speaking, Hannah had, and fortunately regained, a phenomenal memory. She also had, and regained, a sunny personality, a quickness of conversation, and a sharp wit. For a time, these traits were eclipsed as a dark, painful mood disorder blossomed from her injury. Her brain's ability to project her mind was not destroyed, but somehow distorted. This portrait of the many months she spent recovering has much to teach physicians as well as lay readers. The condition she struggled with is neither rare nor trivial, but unfortunately, remains medically unaddressed. Today, in 2014, a patient who has suffered a concussive head injury with minimal structural change can do no more than hope for the best. One day a specific therapy will be at hand.

Bruce Beutler, M.D.

Nobel Laureate, Physiology or Medicine, 2011

CHAPTER 1

IN ONE SPLIT SECOND

January 29, 2012

Jordan and I were on our way to the Torrey Pines golf course for the Farmer's Insurance PGA tournament. Jordan was driving. It was the last day of the tournament and we were excited to watch our friends, Pat Perez and Mike Hartford. Pat was on the leaderboard and Mike was his caddy.

We had just stopped off at Ralph's Grocery Store in the big shopping center across the street from our apartment complex to buy coconut waters. It was a beautiful San Diego morning, eleven a.m. and already seventy-five degrees, not a cloud in the sky. We were leaving the shopping center, first in line waiting for the light to turn green so we could turn left onto the main road, and I realized I was going to be hot. I was wearing a jacket.

"Jordan, I want to go home really quick to change into a short-sleeve shirt," I said.

For an eighteen-year-old, Jordan was well built, a football player. He was also very handsome. People often said he looked like a combination of Tom Cruise and John Travolta. In fact, Jordan had already done a good deal of acting up in Los Angeles, including TV shows on Nickelodeon. It was one of the many things he excelled at.

"No, Mom, we don't have time."

"Jordan, we're going to be out there all day long, I'm going to be so hot."

"No way, come on, we'll be late."

I scowled at him and joked, "Jordan, I would never be married to someone like you 'cause you're so hardheaded."

Without missing a beat, Jordan shot back, "Yeah, well, I'd never be married to someone like you 'cause you're so high maintenance."

Neither of us had any idea how ironic our words were.

The light turned green and Jordan entered the intersection, starting his left-hand turn. Out of the corner of my eye I saw a flash of fluorescent pink, curly hair. It was surreal, like a clown wig. But in a split second I processed that this clown was driving his sedan straight at us; the car was hurtling toward us without braking.

Time slowed down. The next few seconds felt like minutes. I remember staring straight ahead of us at the brick wall across the intersection, thinking, "Oh my gosh, this is it. We're going to die."

The sedan T-boned us, smashing straight into my door at forty-five or fifty miles per hour. I literally felt the sedan hit my right hip. I heard the crash of breaking glass. I had no idea what I hit my head on. In fact, I had no idea I even hit my head. All I felt was the impact from my right knee up to my hipbone, and the violent jarring motion as my head whipped back and forth, left and right. I was wearing my seat belt but my side of the car was crushed and pushed so far in that I ended up basically in Jordan's lap, in the driver's seat. I felt our car skidding across the intersection.

After that, I remember only snapshots as I drifted in and out of consciousness:

Jordan's face was looking at me in terror. "Mom? Mom! Are you okay?"

I already felt the pain in my right hip. I didn't know what had happened to me. But I didn't want to scare him. I remember saying, "Yeah, yeah, I'm okay."

Then I was looking up. But instead of the car ceiling, there was a circle of bright white light. It was like looking into the sun, bright as can be, like a hole of white light surrounded by a field of crystal clear blue.

From a distance I heard Jordan's voice calling me frantically. "Mom? Mom! Come on, we need to get you out of here!"

I was moving towards the white light. It was just like the movies where you see a person leave their body. I was floating upwards, that piercing white circle of light growing larger and larger until it filled my vision. I had just gotten the smallest taste of that light when I suddenly felt myself floating backwards and down again. Words came into my head as if someone spoke directly into my mind.

"It's not your time yet."

The words were vividly clear. It was as if God put those words there, Himself.

Slowly I became aware of my surroundings. The snapshots continued, images fading in and out of darkness as I washed in and out of consciousness.

Jordan was calling to me: "Mom, there's smoke. I smell something burning. We need to get you out of here!"

He was right. I saw smoke in the car. It seemed to be on fire.

Then Jordan was pulling me out of the car.

I found myself standing next to the car, staring at the ground.

"Wait, Mom, I think it's just the radiator. And the dust from the airbags."

I lifted my head slowly and the world started spinning.

Then Jordan was lowering me back down into the driver's seat.

I leaned forward, raised my head, and nausea hit me, hard. Once more everything started spinning. I sat back in the driver's seat again.

Something wet was running down my face. By the look on Jordan's face I knew it had to be blood. I brought my hand up and my face was soaking wet with it.

A blonde woman dressed all in white was suddenly leaning over me, speaking calm words. The way she looked, the way she talked—she was like an angel, peaceful and encouraging. "Sweetheart, it's going to be all right. I called the ambulance. You're going to be okay."

Her name was Brenda. She was trying to keep me conscious. And she was trying to reassure Jordan.

Jordan, though, took complete control of the scene. Once he realized I was safe, he walked over to the sedan to see if the other driver needed help.

Brenda continued speaking to me gently. I drifted in and out. Brenda reclined the driver's seat so I could lay back. She tied something around my head to staunch the flow of blood. Jordan returned to look at me, terribly concerned, but also brave and compassionate. I remember feeling a flash of how proud I was of him.

The next thing I knew there were all these guys in uniforms looming over me, looking down. Paramedics. The ambulance had arrived.

"All right, Hannah," Brenda said. "You're in good hands. I'm going to leave you to them now, honey."

I phased back into consciousness next as the paramedics slipped a board under me in the driver's seat and strapped me down. I heard something about possible head and neck injury.

Then I was in the ambulance. The paramedics were starting to shut the doors.

"Wait! Where's Jordan?"

"It's okay, Miss, just relax, we're gonna get you to the hospital…"

"No! I'm not leaving in this ambulance unless my son comes with me."

I meant it. I wasn't going without Jordan.

Jordan climbed into the ambulance's passenger seat and we took off for the hospital.

I looked down. My jacket was covered in blood. Jordan was trying to reassure me from up front. "You're okay, Mom. You're going to be fine."

A paramedic treated me as we sped along, sirens wailing. The right side of my body was ablaze with pain. The ride was cold, bumpy, and painful. Now my head was hurting. It was worse than anything I had ever felt before, a strange and incredibly intense burning sensation. It literally felt like half my head was on fire. Every bump in the road caused me severe, jarring shocks of pain—and there were a lot of bumps. When, I thought, do they give you something for the pain?

The paramedic, though, was a wonderful man, calm and sweet. He walked me through everything he did. "Okay Hannah, I'm going to put this needle in your arm now for the IV … I know you're cold, Hannah, that's why I'm putting these blankets on you…"

He was right. I was freezing cold and shaking. I had never been in the back of an ambulance before. Wow, I thought, shivering, these things are not very homey. Not a very inviting environment. Everything was cold, clean, and sterile. Which, of course, makes sense. But I couldn't wait to get to the hospital and out of that frigid ambulance.

The paramedic, though, continued being a sweetheart. I remember looking up at him at one point and saying, "You know what? I want to marry someone just like you!"

The next thing I knew they were pulling my stretcher out of the ambulance.

A group of doctors converged on us as we entered the ER. Everyone was talking at once. People were asking my name, details of what had happened. I have no idea what I said.

They brought me straight in for MRI and CT scans to see if there was bleeding on my brain. They locked my head into position with a halo and strapped my body down. I have a memory snapshot of being slid into a freezing cold tube of a machine. I remember being halfway in it and they were talking to me through a little speaker. It was dark and freezing in there.

Quick and clinical, they were trying to do their jobs as fast as possible. Somebody pushed a button and it sounded like a carnival ride revving up. A shrill, frightening, buzzing noise started escalating as the machine wound itself up. It was loud. I didn't really know what was going on, how bad off I was, what was really happening. What was wrong with my head? My hip? My neck? My back? I was phasing in and out of consciousness and scared to death.

Then I was lying in a bed back in the ER, in a little private section of my own with a sheet hanging between the rest of the ER and me. The ER was busy and full. They still hadn't given me anything for the pain. I couldn't believe that. The left side of my head was burning even worse than before, and now it was throbbing as well; electric pulses of agony pounded through my head with every heartbeat. I was crying. The pain in my right hip had spread; now the whole right side of my body felt like it was aflame with red-hot pain. In fact, everything was in pain, every inch of my body. I had no idea which parts of me were injured or not.

A doctor was talking to me, telling me that my BMW saved my life. The other guy's sedan was taller than my 330i and had hit me right in the hip. An eighth of an inch higher and my hip would have been shattered. The right side of my body from my knee to above my waist was one huge, dark bruise from the impact. Now I was feeling pain in my left side too, though. It was internal, the doctor said. My body had been torqued—violently.

Time started straightening out for me a little bit in the ER after the MRI and CT scans. Though still extremely fuzzy, I was more conscious than not. Or, at least, my blackouts were shorter. Jordan stood by me and we went over the events of the accident. He told me about the other driver.

Along with the pink clown hair, Jordan said, this guy's fingernails and toenails were all brightly painted. He had been wearing jean short shorts. It was bizarre. Dolled-up transvestites were not an everyday sight in our quiet little suburban neighborhood. Jordan said that in his driver's license picture he looked like a normal surfer guy. Jordan also said he seemed under the influence of—something. He was in a fog.

It had been a completely clear morning. A Sunday. What had happened? Why did that guy blaze through his red light like that? This clown had had his dubstep music still blaring in his car when Jordan walked over. Jordan actually had to ask him to turn it down.

And then there was no "I'm so sorry—are you okay?" Jordan told me that the only thing this guy said was, "Oh no, I can't believe it! I haven't had an accident in six months!" No remorse whatsoever. No concern for us or our safety. He had plowed through a red light, smashed into us at full speed, here I was in agony in the hospital—and this guy was only worried about his driving record.

Then Jordan's eyes widened and he said, "Mom, do you remember what you said to me right before?"

"Yeah. Well I was right, wasn't I? I hit my head on that damn hard head of yours and look at me!"

The soft part of my head, above my left temple, had hit the hard part of Jordan's head, his forehead. Jordan hadn't tensed during the accident; he hadn't seen the sedan coming. He had just turned his head towards my side of the car when the impact hit.

"Yeah, but Mom, that could've been the last thing you ever said to me!"

We both started laughing like it was the most hilarious joke ever. Of course, I was in shock. It hadn't exactly been a normal day for Jordan either. But it was the truth—Jordan was hardheaded and I was high maintenance. Par for the course.

Jordan called my mom in Tucson. It was too late in the day for her to get to San Diego that night. She would leave first thing in the morning. Then Jordan called my friend, Darrah. We had left our wrecked car at the scene of the accident. We hadn't been there for the police to arrive. We had no idea what was going on with our car, or with whatever it is you have to do, legally, after having a car accident. Basically, we were clueless and carless.

Darrah arrived with her two children. She sat with me in the ER while Jordan came in and out, looking after Darrah's kids in the waiting room. I was glad Jordan got a break from standing watch over me in that busy, bloody ER. I was in terrible pain. Every part of my body hurt worse than anything I had ever felt before, but I knew Jordan couldn't be very comfortable seeing me like this.

Out of nowhere, Darrah said, "Hannah, can I borrow some lip gloss?"

"What? Why?"

"Every one of these male nurses is gorgeous. I guarantee you, in the shape you're in, they're not looking at *you* that way. So can I borrow your gloss?"

It was amazing, given the agony I was in, how hard I laughed at that.

A doctor came in and said he had to staple my head. Darrah left the room.

"Wait!" I said as he approached me. "I work on camera. Don't shave my head! And look—I have an extension right here, don't cut it. Apart from that, you can do whatever you want to me."

He stared at me for a second, not amused. Then he just pulled my hair back and shot that staple gun straight into my head. *BAM-BAM-BAM-BAM-BAM-BAM!* I heard every staple crunch into my head, six times, and each one was excruciating. No warning, nothing to numb me. And then he left. Oh my gosh, I thought, I was such a diva to him that he just slammed those things in, no empathy whatsoever!

Darrah returned and I gave her hell about leaving me. She had thought I wanted some privacy.

They took me in right after that to do a full body X-ray to see if anything was broken in my hip—or anywhere else. The way I was feeling, I would not have been surprised if half the bones in my body had been broken. I was wrapped up like a mummy, with blood all over the gauze on my head.

All the scans came back clear. Darrah, Jordan, and I all breathed sighs of relief. Things settled down. It seemed like nothing major was wrong with me.

After a few more hours they said I could go home. They gave me some pain medication and told me to come back in a week or two so they could remove the staples. On the way out, a doctor told me that the only way for brain injuries to heal was to rest.

Brain injury? Okay. So, I have a brain injury? What does that mean? But they had sent me home with no other instructions than to get some rest, and with nothing more than a bottle of painkillers. So it can't be that bad, right? I must have been very lucky.

Darrah and Jordan brought me home and put me to bed. More than anything I was relieved that Jordan wasn't hurt. I was thankful for that.

I remember lying there in my bed, so grateful, thinking: Jordan's okay. And I'm going to be all right. All this pain—but it was okay. We're alive. It could have been so much worse.

I settled in to get my rest. I could already feel sleep coming.

Everything will be back to normal soon, I thought.

I'll be back to work in a week.

CHAPTER 2

THE FIRST TWO WEEKS

January 30 – February 12, 2012

I awoke the next morning, Monday, January 30, in tremendous pain. My head still felt like it was on fire, though not as bad as the night before. I was taking the pain medication they had given me at the hospital. I hate taking pills and try to avoid them whenever possible, but in this case I knew I needed them. My right side, from my knee to my hip, was still one big ugly black bruise. My left side seemed to hurt even worse—the result, the doctors had told me, of the violent torqueing my insides had suffered.

The pain was terrible. Every small movement of my body set off shockwaves of pain. Jordan left for school and I stayed in bed until Mom arrived later that morning. It was great to see her. My mom and I have always enjoyed a very close relationship. I respect and honor her as much as anyone in this world. Mom had been a hospice nurse for many years and now worked as a massage therapist.

Since the ER doctors had released me only with instructions to rest, I didn't feel the need to visit my regular doctor. But I wanted an adjustment right away to try and get things back in place, so Mom drove me to my chiropractor.

The accident had taken place in the intersection between my apartment complex and the shopping center across the street. As Mom drove us up to that intersection, anxiety hit me. I started sweating. It was very traumatic to sit at that light, thinking back to the accident the day before. I literally started shaking. I was all pins and needles, swiveling my head around, frightened, looking in each direction. I half expected a car to come out of nowhere and cream us.

Mom noticed. She drove very carefully and did her best to calm me, but it was a very intense emotional experience for me to be in a car at all, never mind the fact that the accident had taken place basically right outside my door.

After I told my chiropractor about the accident and the head and neck pain I was feeling, he took X-rays. He told me I was suffering extreme whiplash and had several slipped discs, then he treated me.

Mom got me home after the chiropractor appointment. I was exhausted and went straight to sleep. That day and the next, I was very emotional. I found myself crying at the drop of a hat—which was extremely unusual for me. I was permanently fatigued, sleeping about fourteen hours per day. I would sleep for a few hours, wake up, and try to get out of bed, but the physical pain was overwhelming—my head, neck, back, hips… I'd stay in bed and, before I knew it, I'd be out again, asleep. I spent most of those first two days in bed.

Jordan was great. He did all the chores around the house and gave me the space I needed to rest.

Mom was a huge help too. I didn't have much of an appetite, but Mom was there with soups and juices, trying to get something in me. After the first two days, it seemed like I was getting better and able to do things for myself. It felt like I was on the mend. Mom went home to Tucson but said she'd come right back if I needed her.

I had no car; of course, my BMW was totaled. I needed to get into a rental car. I also needed to get a police report and figure out what was happening, insurance-wise, with the accident. It was the end of the month and all my bills were coming due. As a working single mom, I didn't have much in the way of savings. Missing even a few days of work was difficult financially. Everything came down on me at once. It very quickly started feeling overwhelming.

As the next few days passed, the physical pain slowly decreased. I took less and less of the pain medications during that first week and started feeling better, physically. Still, though, I was sleeping twelve to fourteen hours per day. The only way for a brain injury to heal, they had told me in the ER, was to rest. So it seemed okay to be sleeping so much.

Lying in bed, between sleeping, I often thought back to the moment of impact. It was terrifying. I kept reliving the accident, feeling the crash, seeing some of the snapshots of memory I retained. I would start shaking and sweating, and I would end up lying there in bed, crying, until I fell asleep again.

I also kept remembering that bright white light I had seen in the car, immediately after the accident. The vision of that light and the memory of those words coming into my head—"It's not your time yet"—haunted me. The white light and words didn't exactly scare me—but they kept coming back.

Darrah drove me to the rent-a-car place about a week after the accident. It wasn't easy mustering the energy to get there, but Darrah was a sweetheart and a tremendous help. Once I signed the paperwork, Darrah left me there with my rental car. Getting behind the wheel was very traumatic. As I started driving home, every beep and street noise made me cringe. I would tense my body, waiting for the impact of the accident. And then, halfway home, I suddenly heard a loud *POP!*

I nearly jumped out of my skin. I pulled the car over to the side of the road, trembling and breathing frantically. Finally I got out, looked around at the car, and I couldn't believe it. I was already in this trauma state to be behind the wheel of a car at all and now—on the way home my rental car's tire blew! I texted Darrah. She couldn't believe it.

While I was waiting for someone from the rent-a-car place to arrive, Jordan called me to say that his engine had just blown. Now he was carless. What luck! It was like some kind of dark comedy. It felt like I just needed to stay away from cars completely.

A week had passed since the accident, but I was still spending most of my time in bed. The staples in my head burned and itched. My head was still wrapped in gauze and it would get bloody. I had to change it a few times a day. To unwrap that bloody gauze and stare at my bleeding head, the staples, the bruising and discoloration—it was awful.

I started feeling what I can best describe as "emotionally tired." I continued to cry a lot. I was also constantly listless and fatigued. I would get out of bed, take a few steps, and feel like I had run a marathon. The result was that I didn't want to get out of bed at all. I'd wake up after a few hours of sleep, stand up, feel exhausted, and just go back to bed.

Though the physical pain had diminished during the first week or so, and it wasn't as bad as it had been during the first two days following the accident, it still came and went. And now I was struck with terrible headaches. I did my best to not take the pain meds—I have always preferred to try alternate means of pain reduction rather than taking pills—but the headaches were severe and debilitating.

My close girlfriend, Susanne, who had initially introduced me to Bikram yoga a couple years earlier, suggested I get back into it to help with my physical pain. Bikram is best known as being "the hot yoga." The rooms are brought up to about 105 degrees with high humidity while students go through poses and breathing exercises. I dragged myself there, even though it was very hard to get behind the wheel.

I fought with moments of great indecision when I was driving. I would second-guess myself. I would see a car coming from way down the road and say to myself, "Can I make it in time? Should I go?" And by the time I stepped on the gas to make the turn, I would have waited a bit too long. I probably created some very dangerous situations for myself and other drivers because of that indecision.

Worse, I had to drive through the accident intersection every time I left my house, and it was very traumatic. I would still shake and sweat just sitting in that intersection. I really should not have been driving at all. But I needed something to help with the pain.

I got myself to Bikram and told my instructors about my situation. The studio was called Bikram La Jolla. The owner, Colleen, was a very sweet, very caring woman. She kept an eye on me. Earlier, on the phone, my mom had been amazed when I told her I wanted to try to get back to Bikram. After all, I still had the staples in my head. But I wanted to start building my body back and relieve my pain. Ultimately, Mom believes people should listen to their bodies so she didn't object too much and in fact, the Bikram was a big help. The workout was ninety minutes of hell, but then I had physical relief for a day and a half afterward. When it comes to treatment, I'm a pragmatist. If something works for you—do it. I continued with Bikram because it was effective.

Still, I mostly remember that first week and a half after the accident as being filled with fatigue, pain, and crying. And lots of sleep, day and night. Sometimes I would wake up in the middle of the day, crying, and think back to the morning just a few weeks earlier when I had hiked up a high, steep hill in the Torrey Pines State Preserve. It had been a strenuous climb but I was rewarded with a stunning view overlooking the Torrey Pines golf course, with the ocean sparkling behind it. I sat on a boulder and felt like I was on top of the world. I was in great shape. Everything was going so well. I was invigorated, ready for anything. It felt like nothing could stop me.

Now I was constantly in pain and could barely drag myself out of bed.

About ten days after the accident I started noticing troubling memory-related issues. I was sitting in our living room one of the few times I was actually awake and wanted to ask Jordan to bring me a glass of water. I turned to him and said, "Would you... would you...?"

and I couldn't finish the sentence. I knew I wanted a glass of water, but I just did not have the word for it. The same thing happened as I was looking down at my laptop. I knew the computer was a computer. But I simply could not pull the word "computer" from my memory. It was frightening, but I chalked it up to my fatigue. With more rest, like they had told me, things would be okay. I was just tired.

Since I rented my chair in the hair salon, when I didn't work there was no money coming in—and I still had to pay for the chair. Some of my clients were absolute angels during those first few weeks. They would show up at the house, leave bags of groceries or fully prepared meals by the door—and then just leave. It was a blessing but still, my finances were a mess.

I went back to work about ten days after the accident. I really didn't have a choice, financially. I remember working on one of my first clients. She was sitting in the chair, asking me something about the accident. I stared at her in the mirror, trying to grasp what it was she had asked—and I just couldn't. I couldn't process what it was she had said. It was a completely new feeling for me. It was startling and scary. I knew she was asking something about the accident, and I wanted to reply, but I just stood there with a blank stare on my face. I wanted to speak, but I wasn't really sure of what she had said. And I just couldn't get anything at all to come out of my mouth. I felt disoriented.

Again, it was frightening, but I shook it off as fatigue.

I quickly realized, though, that I could not be on my feet very long. I went into work for only a couple hours at a time. I would take one client and then I'd be exhausted and have to go home.

I was in there doing a highlight one of those days when I suffered my first real episode of overstimulation. I was working on my client's hair when I started becoming very aware—too aware—of all the noises going on around me. Every individual sound started getting very loud in my ears. The blow dryers, the clicking of the curling irons, the people talking … even the music playing in the background started grating on me. I felt anxiety coming on and it quickly progressed to panic. I felt it happening and thought to myself—I'm having a panic attack. I stopped what I was doing and ran outside to take a deep breath.

My client was very sweet about it. When I calmed down a little and walked back inside, she told me to just go home and not worry about it. "Here, Hannah," she said, "I have a Xanax. You should take this and just go home."

I barely finished her highlight, washed her hair, and got her out the door. I didn't cut or dry her hair. I went straight home.

A day or two later I drove myself to the ER. I was still having the headaches. Though it wasn't as severe as the first few days after the accident, I was still in pain. I had had these scary moments of not being able to find the words for things, and now I was feeling overstimulated in everyday situations.

What was wrong with me?

It was about time for the staples in my head to come out so, first thing, the ER doctor removed them. Then, after speaking with me about the pain I was still feeling, he gave me another MRI.

Back into that cold, metal tube. But nothing came back as obviously wrong with me, physically.

As I was leaving the ER, I told the doctor about how I wasn't able to recall words, and about how I had panicked in the salon, feeling overstimulated. A nurse overheard, printed something out, and told me to read it. It said: "post-concussion syndrome." I read it right there.

"Oh my gosh," I said to her, "I had no idea—this is exactly what's happening to me." Right there were the symptoms I had been experiencing: anxiety, sensitivity to light and noise, nausea, disorientation, headaches, irritability, mood swings, short-term memory problems…

The ER doctor said, "Well yes, it makes sense since you had a massive concussion."

My mouth fell wide open. "I did?"

"Of course," the doctor said. He explained that any time someone suffers the kind of head trauma I did, there's a concussion. He told me to expect the symptoms on the PCS pamphlet for the next few months.

It was a shock for me. They had never told me anything about a concussion when they treated me in the ER after the accident. I thought to myself, maybe they told me and I forgot, but I asked Darrah about it and she said no, she didn't remember anyone saying anything about a concussion in the hospital. There was nothing about it on the paperwork they gave me when I was released from the ER.

That pamphlet gave me some clarity. It explained the pain I was still feeling, how I had been crying so much since the accident, the memory issues with the word loss, even the disorientation and overstimulation.

After talking about it a bit more, the ER doctor said he thought I should see a neurologist and made a referral.

The loops I had to jump through to get in to see a neurologist were awful. I tried making an appointment that same day and the earliest they could see me was six weeks off. I couldn't wait six weeks. I called more neurologists and heard the same story.

My friends had been telling me that I needed a lawyer to help deal with the accident ever since it happened. I hadn't thought of it myself but suddenly it seemed very important so I found and retained an attorney. Immediately, I was glad I did it. My attorney got me in to see a neurologist right away. He took the lead in making other doctor appointments for me as well. I had no health insurance, so we searched for doctors who would see me on liens. Not all of them would do that, though, so in some cases my attorney fronted the money himself.

The first time I walked into the neurologist's office, I was struck with the fact that everyone in there had blue hair, gray hair, or pink hair. Only me, being the diva that I am, would notice that about their hair color. But I felt like I was in the wrong place. It was comical. The doctor would come out and say, "Ruth… Ruth… Ruth?" and one of these elderly women would finally hear and shuffle through the door into an exam room. In my subsequent visits, though, that neurologist's waiting room would actually make me feel very fortunate. I saw young kids who had had skateboarding accidents, as well as adults whose bodies were mangled from motorcycle accidents. Those future visits reaffirmed for me that things could always be worse. On this first trip, though, it was just a little funny that I was probably the only one in there under the age of eighty-five.

During that first visit, the neurologist sat me down and explained that brain injuries were very complex. No two were the same. "My job," the neurologist said, "is to watch you. Make sure you're okay. All you can do is rest."

It wasn't closure, it didn't feel like a "real" diagnosis and course of treatment—just having my doctor "watch" me—but it was something. At least I knew now that I had had a concussion. And I was newly aware of something called PCS—post-concussion syndrome. I did research online; I Googled PCS and read whatever I could find. So at least there was a reason for these emotional and memory issues. I wasn't insane, and I wasn't alone. But I also wasn't finished coming down with new symptoms.

I started experiencing extreme ear and jaw pain. It was terrible. It was so intense that I started having a hard time sleeping. My attorney made me an appointment with an ear, nose, and throat specialist who diagnosed me with TMJ—temporomandibular joint disorder. The ENT doctor made me a mouth guard to hold my jaw in place as I slept. It helped, and I was able to get more sleep, but the ear and jaw pain continued. I felt it whenever I was awake—which just made sleeping all the more welcome to me.

I pulled myself into the salon a few more times the second week following the accident. I vividly remember seeing a client of mine, a very kind man named Bruce. He was one of the last clients I was able to work on at the salon. Bruce was a research doctor, an immunologist and geneticist. In fact, Bruce had won the 2011 Nobel Prize in Medicine for his work on immunity. That was pretty amazing, but what really mattered to me was that Bruce was simply a kindhearted man and wonderful friend. I had been doing his hair for years.

As Bruce was paying and leaving the salon, he asked me how I was feeling. He knew about my accident.

"I'm okay," I said, "but I'm still feeling a lot of pain."

Bruce stopped and looked at me kindly.

"Hannah," he said, "it's going to get worse before it gets better."

CHAPTER 3

THE NEXT TWO WEEKS
February 13 – February 27, 2012

A few days later Jordan drove me to Walmart. We grabbed a cart, entered the store, and walked down the first aisle. We hadn't put a single item into our cart when I started feeling overstimulated. It felt like the fluorescent lights were growing brighter and brighter, their harsh light bearing down on me as if they had actual weight. There were too many things on the shelves, too many people crowded around me. My heart started racing. It was as if I could hear every scrape of every shopping cart, every piece of every conversation around me, all of them way too loud. The clothes, the boxes, the shoppers, the lights— it was like being at a stadium rock concert with flashing lights, a crush of humanity, and a barrage of sound, all of them battering my senses. My pulse pounding in my ears, I swiveled my head around, the anxiety growing into a full-blown panic attack. I thought for sure I would have a complete meltdown right there in the store and somebody would call an ambulance. All I could think was, I have to get out of here. We hadn't been in there for more than a minute or two before I had to run outside.

Jordan called after me but I just got out of there. Outside, in the parking lot, Jordan caught up, looked at me like I was crazy, and said, "Mom, you are so weird."

I had driven myself to the grocery store a few times in the previous couple weeks, but I had recently started forgetting what I was there for. On the phone, my mom encouraged me to write lists. I felt like I was ninety years old. After the Walmart experience, though, I started sending Jordan to the store with my credit card. And thank God for the Internet and online bill payments. The few times Jordan and I did go out together after our Walmart trip during those second two weeks after the accident, it happened again, the overstimulation. At least Jordan had seen it happen in Walmart and started understanding when he saw me panicking.

Previously, before the accident, I had gotten into the habit of shooting and uploading daily inspirational videos. Just something to help people get through the day, some positive thought or quote to lift people up and help them face the day with a smile and a proactive attitude. I had worked on-camera as an online webisode host. I got into it while Jordan was working as an actor. Some people who worked in casting told me they thought I would be good on camera as well so I tried it—and I loved it. I took a hosting class and then, together with a friend, I created an online fashion and style show called "Sanctuary of Style." Over the course of about a year we posted twenty episodes on YouTube and other video hosting sites. I also did a few episodes of my own show called "Hair with Hannah" where I would shoot little three-minute tips for women on how to style their hair. Quick and easy "Mom do's" for busy women to look and feel their best. I've always been very social. I love people. I love the Internet webisode format because I can do the videos myself and reach the masses. Everything I did, host-wise, was about helping people look and feel their best.

Into the third week after the accident, I still couldn't do anything as complex as shoot and upload one of those types of webisodes. But I missed doing my daily inspirational videos. So I shot a few. I kept them real short, under a minute. Even that quickly became too much for me, though, and I shortened them to one-line sound bites.

I look back at those videos now and cringe. I am completely "brain-damage girl." I look like a drug addict. I'm standing there, looking like I had been up for a week straight, dazed, searching for words, stuttering… I have since given Jordan and my friends all kinds of hell about it—"How could you let me post those?!"

Pretty soon, though, I couldn't even do those one-line sound bites. Shooting them was too overstimulating. Right around the third and fourth weeks after the accident, it got to the point where I could hardly stand to hear any sound at all.

Jordan would come home from school, find me in bed, and start talking to me, excited to share his day. It would be too much for me.

"Jordan, please, you have to keep it down. I can't handle it, please."

"Come on, Mom, I just want to tell you what happened…"

"Jordan, really, please! Can you please keep it down?"

"Mom! I'm not talking loud!"

Poor Jordan only wanted to share, like he had on a daily basis with me before the accident. But I couldn't bear it.

I started missing doctor's appointments. I had driven myself to a few, but driving was so traumatic that I had had instances where I just pulled the car over to the side of the road and cried and cried. The memory of the accident would come rushing back. I was off the pain medication but I was still, somehow, just not coherent.

I barely had the energy to walk to the toilet never mind shower, dress, and drive myself to the doctor… even the thought of it was exhausting.

I started sliding down a slippery slope. I couldn't function. I couldn't leave my room. Any light or sound was overstimulating to my brain. I would literally crawl from my bed to the bathroom. I had zero energy and always felt physically fatigued. I experienced double vision—periodically images would double up and streak and run together, as if I was drunk. Oftentimes I just couldn't answer the phone. The voices were too loud. I couldn't watch TV—the movement on-screen, the flashing lights, the noise—it was too much.

Over the phone, my mom started noticing that things were getting worse. I wouldn't retain what she said, even right after she said it. I think "What?" was my favorite word during those weeks. I asked her to repeat basically everything she said to me. I called her crying sometimes, telling her about the appointments I was missing. I still didn't have a police report, I was still dealing with the insurance company, everything was in limbo, and everything seemed completely insurmountable.

I was absolutely overwhelmed. Mom would make lists for me over the phone. She told me to make my days doable. I would be anxious about all the things I needed to get done, overwhelmed with the big picture, and she'd say, "Hannah, bring it back to right now, this minute. What can you handle now? Forget about whatever you're supposed to do today. What one thing do you think you can handle just now?" It was great advice, to break my errands and responsibilities down to little pieces. But the truth is, I couldn't even handle that. Focusing on anything at all was an unbearable chore. Mom saw that and came back to help.

Still, she didn't know how bad things were until she arrived. I reverted back to being like a child. I would snuggle up to my mom on the couch and talk to her like I was a little kid. "Mom? Mommy?" I was very much in need. I couldn't take care of myself. And I had a child of my own. It felt just terrible.

Mom bought a juicer for me. I had no appetite and I couldn't handle sitting down to a full meal. Just looking at a plate of food and thinking about the process of eating it made me feel like going back to bed. Mom was able to get nutrients into me with that juicer. And sometimes she sat on my bed and fed me like I was a toddler. Mom is big on drinking lots of good, clean water, so she provided that for me as well. If she hadn't been there offering me glass after glass, I doubt I would have drunk any, myself, during those days.

Mom brought me to my doctor appointments. A few days into her visit, toward the end of week three, I tried driving, with Mom in the passenger seat. We were on the way to my chiropractor and I had a complete meltdown on the freeway. Everything got loud and bright; the cars on either side of me kept feeling like they were going to crash into me. I pulled off the freeway, slammed the car into park—and started sobbing. I used to drive back and forth to Los Angeles from San Diego all the time. I couldn't believe this was happening to me. Mom knew I shouldn't have been driving; she had tried to talk me out of it. I was trying to be stubborn and independent. The whole situation was depressing and confusing—one step forward, two steps back.

It was a huge chore for me to get my bills together. Mom helped me organize my finances—and they were a wreck. Just because Mom helped me put my bills in order didn't mean I had the money to pay them though. Friends and family had made gifts of money to me. That was hard to take. I have always been fiercely independent. It has always been me helping other people out, not the other way around. I've been the glue in my family, keeping us together, updating my brothers and my mom on what everyone else was doing. I was the one who would help out whenever someone needed it.

But now I was the one needing the help. It was a lesson in humility. Still, it wasn't nearly enough. The power company came out to shut off our electricity while my mom was there. This guy was literally at the door, telling us he was going to turn off the electricity. I started freaking out. Mom told me not to worry. She was able to give the power company guy just enough money to keep the power on. For now.

My daily living activities were completely compromised. I couldn't shop, cook, pay my bills—I couldn't even feed myself.

On the third or fourth Sunday morning after the accident, Mom and Jordan came into my room.

"Hannah," Mom said, "we're going to church now. Would you like to come?"

My faith has always been completely solid and extremely important to me. I wanted to go very badly but just couldn't muster the energy.

"No, Mom."

"Mom!" Jordan said. "Come on, just go to church with us. It'll be good..."

I exploded. "Fuck you! Fuck you and fuck church! Get out of here, leave me alone!" I was lying in my bed, screaming at them. I'll never forget the look on Jordan's face. He had no idea what was going on, why I was acting this way. My faith has always been so strong. They just shut the door and slinked away.

It was like I had Turret's. I stayed in bed all day, crying.

A few days later Mom was cooking a pot of soup. I had agreed to do her hair so I dragged myself out of bed and shuffled into the kitchen. Jordan was in the living room nearby, watching TV.

The dishwasher was going. It started pounding in my ears. The soup was bubbling on the stove in a way that made my stomach turn. There were groceries on the counter and somehow they seemed so jumbled and confusing. The overhead light felt way too bright, the TV was blaring in my ears; everything was just—too much. I started sweating and getting dizzy, like I was standing on a cliff. I saw my mom staring at me. She asked me what was wrong. I said something about it being too loud in the kitchen, too noisy, too many things going on at one time. From the couch Jordan said, "Come on, Mom, it's not that noisy..."

I snapped. I don't know what I screamed but whatever it was, it was loud and it was rude. I ran back to my room, slammed the door, curled up into a ball on the bed, and cried hysterically. I was in there like that for two hours.

When I finally gathered the strength to come out, I went to my mom, crying, saying, "Mom, I'm sorry, I'm so sorry, I feel like I'm crazy..."

Mom did her best to soothe me, hugging me, calmly repeating, "It's okay, honey, you're not crazy, it's okay…"

BUT REALLY I WAS CRAZY.

Mom had never seen me act anything like this. I was used to chaos in my house. I have a teenage boy. I'm used to having the house filled with big, loud high-school football players. I'd be cooking, joking, texting—I am the queen of multitasking. Or, I was.

This was all so foreign to me.

Some days were better, some were worse. It was beyond frustrating that these second two weeks after the accident were actually worse, emotionally and mentally, than the first two weeks.

But with Mom's help I did get better at breaking my days into doable tasks. I got better at not letting the big picture engulf me. I made lists. Sometimes there was literally one item on my list, but it helped me keep things in perspective and not get overwhelmed.

With Mom and Jordan tending to me, I started regaining my strength toward the end of the fourth week. I started cooking for Jordan and feeding myself. I started functioning. It felt like things were getting better so we all figured Mom could go back home.

Before she left, Mom had a talk with me. She used to work as a hospice nurse. She told me that what I was going through was really a grief process. I needed to process what had changed in my life and how things were going to be different, moving forward. I had to accept that things had changed. I had changed. I had a "new normal," she told me.

Honestly, I didn't know what was normal for me anymore. And I had no idea what things were going to be like in the future. Mom had seen me at my worst now. She had seen me blow up, curse, shout, freak out, and cry in my room hysterically for hours. But with Mom's encouragement I did start accepting that things were going to be different. I wasn't sure exactly how—but they would be different. The doctors had said we needed to wait a year, and then see where I was. There was no way to tell how different, how changed, I would be, permanently. It was very frightening.

But Mom was there to say, "It's okay, Hannah. Whatever happens— it'll be okay." And she told me over and over how much she loved me.

I didn't know where I was going to end up, but I knew I was loved. And I knew that wherever I ended up, somehow, it was going to be okay. With those words, Mom gave me the greatest gift. She gave me the grace to get through each day.

CHAPTER 4

THE NEXT TWO MONTHS

March – April 2012

After a total of two weeks, Mom went back to Tucson. Again, I had regained much of my strength and seemed better able to take care of myself. And again Mom said if I needed her, she'd come right back.

I tried working at the salon a few more times in early March, but it became increasingly difficult. I'd be exhausted after an hour on my feet, and I continued to feel overstimulated by the sights and sounds at the salon.

I was off the pain meds completely but still wasn't coherent. Driving still caused me great anxiety—every sound from the road made me tense up, awaiting a collision. And I had to pass through that intersection where the accident had taken place every single time I left my house, reliving the trauma of the accident every single day, if not multiple times per day.

I would arrive at places and then forget why I was there and how I got there. I started missing my doctor appointments again— lots of them.

I could have asked Mom to return, but she had sacrificed so much to come out twice already. Honestly, though, I was sick of talking about my injuries and recovery. It felt like every time I opened my mouth I was complaining. Nobody likes to hear that all the time. I was sick of it, myself. I wanted to give my mom a break. She had her own life.

Jordan started noticing cognitive changes in me. A few years earlier I had developed the habit of reading the dictionary. I encouraged Jordan to expand his vocabulary as well and would intentionally use "big words" with him. Now, though, reading anything became a chore. I used to keep a couple self-help books by my bed. I was always reading one or two of them. Now I just couldn't focus. I could barely get through a doctor's bill, never mind a page of the dictionary.

I would reread everything several times, trying to process the words. I couldn't seem to hold things in my memory the way I had before. By the time I processed a new sentence, I would forget what I had read just a sentence or two earlier. While speaking, I still struggled to find the simplest words—they eluded me, like I couldn't access parts of my brain the way I used to. Jordan joked that I didn't sound as "smart" as I used to.

Humor was actually a big part of our communication. It had to be. If I didn't laugh about all these changes, I would just cry. Still, though, to hear that from Jordan made me wonder just when all this would be behind me. And not just "when," but—"if." Would I ever sound "smart" again? I had no idea.

I lost a good deal of my sense of taste and smell. I would find myself adding salt to taste. I'd taste something, add salt, taste it, add more salt—and then I would realize: I never add salt to my food. As a high school football player, Jordan's room used to have a certain, shall we say, olfactory presence to it that would make me sometimes cringe as I passed his door. I have always had a supersensitive nose. Now, though, I wouldn't have smelled Jordan's feet if he had rubbed them in my nose right after football practice.

Financially, I was drowning. Jordan and I used to go on date nights. We would go to dinner or the movies regularly. I told Jordan I was training him to be the perfect husband. Those outings had to stop, though. Everything nonessential was eliminated—and there wasn't nearly enough for the essentials.

Again, though, humor helped. I would be sitting on the couch and look over at Jordan with a blank stare and say, "Excuse me? Who are you and why are you sitting on my couch, eating all my food?" Sometimes I'd look at him, out of the blue, shake my head, and say, "You know what, I know I'm supposed to be stressing out about something but I can't remember what it is… oh yeah—rent is due tomorrow and I'm seven hundred dollars short!" We'd laugh. But it was true! That "joke" regarding the rent happened several times—for real. I would know I should be worrying about something but I'd forget what it was. In a way, that forgetfulness was a blessing at times. I didn't always know how bad things were!

On April 1, I gave up my chair at the salon. The rent was $1,500/month. I couldn't handle the stimulation at the salon anymore. I wasn't going in, so it didn't make sense to pay the rent on my chair. But it meant giving up even the illusion that I would be making a living there at the salon.

I missed doing hair. It was a great creative outlet for me, but more importantly it was something that brought true joy to my spirit. I was able to, literally, transform people. I've always said that if your hair isn't working, nothing is. It all starts at the top. Then come the makeup and clothes. I used to love watching people stand up from my chair. They would walk taller. They would have a big, genuine smile on their face. They would feel better about themselves and that made me feel fantastic. It brought me instant gratification, building people's confidence. I became very close to my clients. I treated them the way I'd like to be treated. I have always loved people and getting to know them. A lot of beans were spilled in my chair, a lot of secrets shared. I believe that when people feel bad, they usually phone either their doctor or their hair stylist. Clients would call to book an appointment and tell me they needed their "Hannah time." And then they'd say, "Oh yeah, and we need to do my hair too!"

My clients loved what I did with their hair—but they told me that the talks we had were even more important to them. Losing that feeling of helping people was something that meant quite a bit to me.

During those weeks I continued to spend most of my time in my bedroom. I was still sleeping twelve to thirteen hours a day—and feeling like I hadn't slept at all. I remained constantly fatigued and exhausted. During the day I'd be up for an hour, then asleep for two. I didn't want to eat. I didn't want to shower. I didn't want to face the bills. I just wanted to sleep.

Jordan would walk in after school and I'd have the windows closed, the drapes drawn. We'd repeat our pattern: he'd start telling me about his day and I'd tell him he was being too loud. He'd tell me I wasn't paying attention, that I didn't care. I'd put my hands over my ears and tell him I just couldn't handle the noise. Jordan would leave, peeved, telling me I had a bad attitude.

One day in mid-March Jordan walked in, looked around, and told me it was depressing in my room. That set me off. I denied it. I told him he didn't understand what it was like for me. I told him I wasn't depressed, I just needed my sleep—that's what the doctors had told me; the only way for the brain to heal is to sleep. Hence the dark, quiet room. Jordan didn't mention it again. I have to admit, I'm sure that for Jordan, simply walking into my room was like playing with fire. We argued a lot in those days, over the smallest things.

I was unable to push Jordan, positively, the way I always had in the past. I could barely function, barely take care of my own basic needs. Jordan was doing the shopping and most of the chores. In the past I had made a point to always stay on his case about being productive. I encouraged him to use his time wisely. A day off from school wasn't an invitation to sit on the couch all day. Jordan had a tendency to procrastinate so I often needed to prod him into doing his homework.

Jordan's grades started slipping and I didn't have a clue—until I got a call from his school. I was very upset and let Jordan have it. But what I didn't tell him was how upset I was with myself. It felt terrible. I wasn't able to be that positive voice anymore, pushing my son to do his best.

I kept a written journal. My doctors had asked me to, to keep track of my symptoms and behavior. It was a very good idea in retrospect. Since my memory was so bad, if I hadn't kept that journal I would have forgotten everything that happened. In those days the entries were all basically the same:

Another day in bed. Migraine headache. Mentally clouded. Pain in my shoulders. Emotional. Crying. And still not retaining any information. Can't even focus to fill out paperwork. Waking up with pain. Anxiety. Left leg and hip in extreme pain...

I continued seeing my chiropractor for the hip pain but I missed more appointments than I made.

I missed my friends greatly. I would lie in bed and think: as social as I am—how could I not even be able to go out in public? I had always loved meeting new people. All my life, it had been one of my greatest assets and joys. I took pride in it, being able to go out for coffee and come back with a phone number and a new friend. All of a sudden it was like—I'm an introvert now? I never understood what being an introvert was or meant. Now I was living it.

April 11 is a day I won't forget. Jordan came home from football practice. As usual, I was in bed and as usual Jordan came in to share his day with me. Immediately, he was talking way too loud for me.

"Jordan, keep it down."

"Mom, I'm not being loud. I lost my wallet. I know I'll find it but..."

"Really, you can't talk this loud. Keep it down. I can't retain what you're saying."

"Mom, come on. You're fine. Just get out of bed. It's all in your head."

I don't think I ever moved so quickly in my life. I leaped out of that bed and started screaming: "You get out of my house! You don't understand! You are disrespecting me!"

And then I started choking my son. I had him around the throat with both of my hands and I was literally choking him, yelling, "You don't know what I'm going through! You get out of my house! Get the hell out!"

I did it. I took his phone and his car keys, I kicked him out of the house, and I locked the doors.

I ran back to bed. My heart was pounding. I was so worked up, so anxious, I thought about calling an ambulance. I was shaking and sobbing.

Then I heard, "Mom? Mom?" I ran into the living room. Jordan was crawling through a window, trying to get back inside, but he was stuck halfway in.

"Mom! Don't do anything crazy!" There was fear in Jordan's eyes. He knew, at that moment, that I was capable of anything. For all he knew, given the scene I had just made, I was going to run into the kitchen, grab a knife, and attack him as he was stuck there in the window. He was pleading with me. "It's okay, Mom, stay calm, I just want to grab a few things, then I'll go, it's okay..."

Jordan got himself inside, quickly packed some clothes into a suitcase, and left. I sent him into the street with no cell phone and no car.

Then I spent the night crying in bed.

The next morning I felt absolutely terrible. Never in a million years would I have thought, in the past, of kicking Jordan out of the house. We had always been able to talk our way through things. We were, in fact, best friends. I had never raised a hand to my son in my life. But last night I had grabbed him by the throat and squeezed. The one thing I had never wanted to do to my son was kick him out of the house. I had *never* wanted to be that kind of parent. It was against all of my beliefs. Jordan had been doing all the chores, the shopping, the errands. He shouldn't have had to deal with all this. He was supposed to be enjoying his senior year in high school. I was robbing him of that.

And I felt robbed, myself, of being present for it, sharing it with him, participating. I was supposed to be supporting him. Instead, he was having to take care of me. And now look how I was treating him. It made me all the sadder.

I texted Jordan's girlfriend, asking if he was with her. The answer was yes. As I had expected, Jordan had walked to her house and spent the night. I texted back: *Please tell him I need to talk to him*.

Jordan came home that evening. I apologized. I felt horrible. I told him that he didn't deserve to be treated that way no matter what I was going through. He told me he didn't know what to do—I had looked crazy. In his own words, he told me he "had seen the devil" in my eyes.

Jordan was eighteen years old. He shouldn't be asked to go through this kind of thing.

My mom came back a few days after that. Things were not good in my house, and she could tell.

Mom was able to get me back into the routine of going to my doctor appointments. But those appointments left me very frustrated. The doctors didn't seem to get it. It had been months and I was still spending my days in bed, sleeping more or less around the clock. I was still extremely volatile, emotionally, and in great pain. My doctors would listen and then offer to give me another pain medication. I would say no. The pain meds fogged me up and I was already walking around in a fog all day long as it was. I felt like I needed to be as logical as possible. I would leave those appointments in tears. I was hoping for some new information or treatment, but all my doctors would do was tell me to rest. They would continue to keep an eye on me and wait to see how things developed.

My jaw and neck pain had intensified, so my primary physician referred me to another doctor who would give me something to relax my muscles. It was April 16 and I'll never forget it. This new doctor gave me thirty injections in one sitting, straight into my jaw, ears, neck, and back. It was the most painful thing I have ever experienced in my life. Each shot was agony and they just kept coming, like they were never going to end. I went home, curled up in bed, and cried the entire night.

April 20 was another day I'll always remember, but for a very different reason. I was sitting on the couch with Mom. I had dragged myself out of bed, an act of will, to spend some time with her. We were watching *Ellen* and she was interviewing a movie producer, promoting his new film. This guy had produced and directed, among others, some very successful Jim Carrey movies. Jordan absolutely loves Jim Carrey. This producer's new film, though, was a documentary.

Then the guy started talking about his bicycle accident. He said he had suffered post-concussion syndrome. It had changed his life. He lost everything. It reached the point where he just couldn't be around other people; he couldn't leave his house. The overstimulation had been too much. He stopped functioning and had to move out of his mansion and into a little trailer on the beach.

I sat up on the couch. What?!

His name was Tom Shadyac. He went on to say that, for him, the symptoms had lasted between six months and a year. I'll never forget. Mr. Shadyac took a moment to say, very seriously, something like: "I just want to say… if anyone is suffering from this, I want you to know that you will get better. And at the other end, at the other side of this, things will be okay. In the midst of it, I know, it doesn't feel like it at all but—listen, hang in there, it's going to get better."

I was sitting there with my mouth open. Who the heck is this guy?!

Mr. Shadyac told Ellen that he had found his true purpose as the result of his PCS. Previously he had been making very successful comedies. But now he was spending his time making socially impactful documentaries, writing a book, and doing a variety of charity work. He had reinvented himself. There's absolutely nothing wrong with making the next big Jim Carrey movie, but now this guy was a powerful, positive force, bringing water to drought-stricken areas in Africa and reaching out to people who had suffered PCS—people like me!

Mom and I looked at each other. It was a classic "ah-ha!" moment. I wasn't alone. This is what I've been experiencing, I thought; this is what's been going on with me—the same thing this guy went through. He's on a journey just like mine. And look how positive he's become!

The PCS pamphlet the ER nurse had given me back in February had brought me clarity. It had listed the PCS symptoms and as a result, I was able to put a name on the condition I had been suffering. I had read it to my mom and to Jordan and it gave us some information— but then that pamphlet had gone into my huge file of doctor paper- work. It had explained the signs and symptoms. But it hadn't said that things would actually get worse as the weeks went by. It hadn't said how long the symptoms would last. It had given me a name for what was happening, but it had been a bit like reading the back of a bottle of cold medicine—expect these symptoms—and not much else.

Now I had seen a real person talk about his real experience with PCS. And it was actually inspiring! After hearing Tom Shadyac speak—speak as if he were talking to me, alone—I immediately started Googling PCS, right there on the couch. Everything before had been nebulous and vague. It had been frustrating, suffering these symptoms but not fully knowing and understanding. Seeing Tom Shadyac and hearing him tell about his personal story, it hit me for the first time that others had actually come through the same thing I was suffering—and had become better people on the other side. The one logical thought I had had, ever since the beginning, as I had watched myself going through the emotional turmoil—exploding in anger, crying and sobbing in bed for hours—was: *this isn't me*. This isn't the person I really am.

I watched TV maybe an hour a week in those months. I hardly left my bed and that was all I could take of the flashing lights and loud noise. It was blind luck that Mom and I had flipped on *Ellen* that time. What were the odds that I'd actually be sitting on the couch, not in bed, watching TV, and happen to turn on *Ellen* when this exact guy, Tom Shadyac, was telling his story of living through PCS? They were astounding.

I Googled like a madwoman. I researched PCS extensively. I shared what I found with Mom and Jordan. Jordan read everything I asked him to and started really understanding what was going on with me.

I educated myself and it gave me hope. Frankly, it was like someone had thrown me a lifeline. But it didn't mean the symptoms or the frustrations stopped.

I still needed a new car. The very last thing I wanted to deal with was a car. My attorney was very kind and diligent, but insurance cases like this drag on at a snail's pace. I still didn't have my insurance check for a new car because I just didn't have the strength and focus to finish the paperwork. Mom was a big help but I was extremely limited in what I could handle.

My journal entries continued to be very grim. Still, almost every day I would write something like: *Woke up with a headache. Feeling very emotional. Extremely tired. Crying at the drop of a hat. Not retaining any info. My sciatica pain is extreme. Feel in a fog at all times. I'm feeling very anxious. Physically can't get out of bed. Mentally not sure of my surroundings. I have regressed.*

Writing even that much was a terrible chore. Physically, emotionally, mentally, I was simply overwhelmed. I felt so alone.

I went back for another round of injections on April 26. Thirty more shots, straight into my jaw, ears, neck, and back. It was brutal. The pain was incredible. How long would I have to go through all this? More than anything, I just wanted the pain to stop. I was feeling extremely down. Things were just getting worse.

I remember lying in bed after those injections, crying, a complete wreck, and a single thought struck me: All I want to do is see my son graduate from high school. That was it. That was my only goal in life. After that, I said to myself, I can pass away.

CHAPTER 5

THE OCEAN

April 30, 2012

I woke up on the morning of Monday, April 30, 2012, feeling extremely anguished. I was emotionally distraught and crying. I had stopped journaling. I didn't have the energy or focus to continue writing down every detail of my misery and pain. Nothing changed. Every day it was pain—physical, emotional, and mental. I was a mess.

Jordan was in Santa Barbara for the day. He was planning to attend college there and was taking his placement tests to see which courses he would qualify for.

This morning, the pain in my neck and back was unusually dreadful. I knew I needed to relieve myself of the physical pain somehow. I would either drive myself to the ER or to yoga.

I decided on yoga.

I parked my car outside Colleen's studio, Bikram La Jolla. I sat there and realized that my anguish was accompanied by an inexplicable numbness. I was in terrible pain, physically and emotionally, but I was also miserably detached from everything at the same time. It was like an out-of-body experience. If I had dug a knife into my arm, drawing blood, I don't think I would have even felt it. It felt like part of my brain had flipped a switch and completely shut me off from everyone else in the world. I was in my own lonely universe of pain. I felt completely hopeless. It seemed like all this pain would never stop. Thoughts of hopelessness were drowning me. I'm a burden to others. No one would miss me if I was gone. I can't do it anymore.

I started crying hysterically. I sat in my car sobbing and shaking.

I picked up my cell phone and called my mother. I told her I was in a very bad place, alone and completely despondent.

"Hannah, you need to trust God. He has everything in control. Put yourself in His hands."

Anger spiked inside of me. Through my tears I yelled into the phone, "That's bullshit! Fuck God! If He loved me I wouldn't be here like this!" I hung up on my mom.

It was *not* what I needed to hear. It didn't feel to me like this had anything to do with God. It had to do with me having absolutely no control over my life—my pain.

I was crying uncontrollably. Looking straight ahead, through my windshield, I could see the ocean. A few blocks away, the road ended in a cliff, high over the sea. All I had to do was step on the gas and go. A couple blocks and I could drive straight off the cliff, into the ocean. The pain would be over. The anguish. I'm going to do it, I thought. I'm going to drive my car off that cliff and into the ocean.

I looked down at my phone and—I'm not sure why but—I called Darrah. I was still bawling.

"Hannah? What's going on?"

"I'm going to do it."

"...You are?"

"Yeah."

"Do you know how you're going to do it?"

Darrah knew exactly what I was talking about.

"Yeah."

"Are you going to drive off into the ocean?"

I was silent. It was amazing. She also knew exactly how I was going to do it.

Darrah continued. "Are you at Bikram?"

"Yeah."

"Hannah, you have to think about all the good things in your life, your wonderful family and friends who love you dearly. Life would not be better if you were gone. You would forever wound so many people. Your son is coming home from the train station tonight. You have to pick him up. That's your job. And right now, the one thing you have to do is to grab your yoga mat and walk into Bikram La Jolla. It doesn't matter if you just lie there on your mat for ninety minutes. Just go. And then tonight your one job is to pick up your son. Go. But if you walk back out that door, you call me right away. Do you understand?"

Darrah was with me. Somehow she was right there with me, on my level, speaking my language. I could listen to her.

I closed my eyes through the tears and just said, "Okay, Darrah."

I went in, put down my mat, and lay down. I didn't do any poses. I didn't move. I just lay there, crying. The owner, Colleen, was very understanding and allowed me my space. I'm sure everyone else around me in class was wondering what the hell was wrong with me.

After ninety minutes, when the class finished, I walked out. I was still completely numb, emotionally and physically. I walked down to the beach.

The beach has always been a place of connection for me. I visited the beach often. I would take off my shoes, put my feet into the sand, and let the ions of the ocean ground me. I could always find peace and happiness where the ocean meets the land. The beach has always been a place of great gratitude for me.

This time I walked onto the sand, down to the water, sat down—and I was still completely numb. I looked into the ocean. Nothing. Just numb. I sat there for an hour.

I thought back to what Darrah had said. My job today, the one thing I had to do, was pick up Jordan at the train station. It was a responsibility I couldn't shirk. It was my son. I focused on that, alone.

I don't know how I was able to drive that day but I got myself home, relaxed in bed, and did absolutely nothing until the time came to pick up Jordan.

I drove to the train station. In the car, I shared with Jordan what had happened earlier that day. I needed him to know what was going on with me. I told him I almost took my own life today. It shook him. But Jordan had been growing more and more in tune with what was going on with me over the past weeks and months.

We made it home and I slept nearly around the clock for two days straight. Crippled and paralyzed, I just couldn't get out of bed.

I came out of my room after those two days and sat down next to Jordan on the couch. The news was on. Retired NFL star Junior Seau had committed suicide in his home, nearby, in Oceanside. It was May 2, 2012. He had shot himself in the chest. The reporters were saying that a year earlier he had tried committing suicide by driving his car off a cliff—exactly what I had been planning outside yoga. The reporters also spoke about the possibility that Junior Seau had been suffering concussion-related symptoms including depression. They were speculating that, like Dave Duerson—another NFL player who had shot himself in the chest so that his brain could be studied for brain trauma—Seau may have been hoping that doctors would study his brain to see whether or not there was brain injury as the result of his long and violent football career.

Some people on TV said they thought Junior Seau had acted very selfishly—he had children. How could he take his own life?

All I could think was—I knew exactly how Junior Seau had felt. I had had the exact same plan—driving my car into the ocean. If you have thought your suicide out, and everything is perfectly aligned at that moment, you will follow through with it.

I also knew that that kind of anguish came and went. It's not there all the time. But when it comes, it is very nearly inescapable. Thank God for Darrah and the responsibility of picking up my son.

The coincidence of Junior Seau committing suicide two days after I considered the same thing—both, perhaps, as the result of trauma to the brain and the ensuing personality changes—was like some sort of signpost for me.

My friend, Lauryn, called me later that day. This was another remarkable coincidence. Though Lauryn and I are very close, she never calls. We always text. She called to ask about a hair appointment. She didn't know I had stopped doing hair.

I was still emotionally numb and Lauryn heard it in my voice. Very quickly she said, "Hannah? Is that really you? Oh my God. Everything I hear in your voice is exactly what I heard in my mother's voice right before she committed suicide."

I hadn't told Lauryn what had happened outside yoga two days earlier.

Lauryn's mom had taken her own life when Lauryn was in high school. Her mother had suffered from depression.

I started crying on the phone. I hadn't thought of myself as "depressed." I knew I was in physical pain, I knew I was in mental and emotional anguish—but who really knows what a brain injury does to someone? Every injury is different. Every minute is different and you can't predict what's going to happen next.

"Hannah," Lauryn said, "you need to go to your doctor today, and by two o'clock you better have a pill in your mouth. If you don't, I will come there and physically take you to the doctor and make sure they give you something for depression.

"It's not about you, Hannah," Lauryn continued. "It's not about what type of person you are, how strong you are, what your faith is like—depression is a disease. Just like cancer. You have to treat it. You're not just going to get better by crying. You need medicine. There's something chemically unbalanced in your brain and you need medication."

Because of her mom, I knew that Lauryn knew a lot about

depression. She had researched it extensively. I had no idea I was suffering from depression until Lauryn told me I sounded like her mom. Darrah and Jordan had hinted at it, but I think they were afraid of what my reaction would have been had they truly confronted me about it, given how volatile I was.

I gave Lauryn my word and then called my doctor. I explained how I was feeling. He didn't even need me to come in. He called in a prescription for Zoloft. I've always been an anti pill-popper so this was foreign to me.

Jordan went to the pharmacy to get the prescription for me. I took one pill, twenty-five milligrams. My heart started pounding and racing. The skin was crawling off my body. Oh my God, I thought, *now what?!* I didn't know what was going on, I thought I'd have to go to the ER again.

I called my doctor and he said since I'd never been on this kind of medication before, I should start with ten or fifteen milligrams.

I started taking the lower dosage and within a few days, slowly, it was like the sun was coming out and my eyes were slowly opening to it. I had been walking around in a dark fog. I used to go into Starbucks or the bank, say hello, meet people, and genuinely care. Since the accident I was barely able to say hello to people I knew. I had been leading a sort of flat-lined existence. Taking the Zoloft was like being able to see life again.

I wasn't paralyzed in my bed anymore. And I mean paralyzed quite literally. The thought, just the thought, of lifting my arm had been exhausting. I used to lie there thinking, am I ever going to get my arms up out of this bed again?

The Zoloft cut through the dark membrane separating me from the rest of the world, and that was a very, very big deal. It was a blessing. I started getting myself out of bed and into the car. But it didn't mean I had any real answers.

If I had broken my arm, I would have had a cast put on it and known that within six weeks my bone would be healed and I'd be able to use my arm again. With my brain injury, though, the doctors had only said to wait and see. Well, after three months, things continued to get worse. There was no indication anything was getting better. Just the opposite. It's not visible. You can't see the brain the way you can see your broken arm. You can't see it improve. You don't even know if it's improving at all. All you know is things are getting worse and you can only wonder: will it be like this for the rest of my life?

CHAPTER 6

TWO MORE MONTHS – I'M NOT ALONE / I'M ALL ALONE

May – June 2012

After hearing about my suicidal thoughts outside yoga, Mom came back out again a few days later. Like the previous two times, with Mom there to help, I started making progress. We were able to get me a car. And again, Mom brought me to my medical appointments.

After seeing Tom Shadyac on *Ellen* and researching PCS, I found out that doctors used PET scans to help diagnose brain injuries. I wanted to know for sure exactly what was wrong. I wanted to learn how, specifically, I could help heal myself. But my doctor kept saying that the right course of action was just to continue to wait and see how my symptoms progressed. I remained persistent with my request for the PET scan but he wouldn't order it.

Feeling better, I drove us to one of my chiropractor appointments. Mom tried to talk me out of it but I insisted. It was about a twenty-minute drive. We hadn't gotten far on the freeway when I had a full-blown panic attack. The memory of the accident, the anxiety of being behind the wheel—they overwhelmed me. I started shaking and crying hysterically. Mom had me pull off the freeway as soon as possible. I sat there behind the wheel, sobbing.

It took about twenty minutes for me to calm down. Mom kept

soothing me the whole time, speaking calmly and reassuring me that everything was okay. Her mantra to me, that day and other days, was to forget about the big picture and focus on *now*.

"Don't worry about the chiropractor," she said. "Don't worry about driving. Don't worry about anything. Right now we're in this car, everything is all right, and the only thing you have to do is calm down and remember that everything is okay."

Mom kept telling me to give myself a break. I wasn't the same person I had been before the accident. Things had changed. I wouldn't function the same way. They were the same things Mom had been telling me for months now. In general it was a huge help. But in certain situations, on certain days, the overstimulation still came, the sensory overload, the utter exhaustion, the frustration, the emotional volatility. It wasn't going away.

Still, I pushed myself—or tried to. While Mom was there this visit, one day we decided to spend some time down at my apartment complex's pool. She gathered towels and waters for us and we left the apartment. Immediately I started feeling tired. We hadn't even reached the pool when I felt so incredibly fatigued that I had to turn around, go back inside, and crawl into bed.

Mom did her own research regarding alternative treatments for brain injuries. She had a friend who had suffered brain trauma. This friend told Mom how beneficial a treatment called cranial sacral work had been for her. Mom found a woman who performed this treatment nearby and offered to pay—if I was onboard to try it, she said, she didn't want money to stand in the way. I agreed.

The session included this woman placing her fingers on my head in various spots, barely touching me. I was lying there, comfortably, and suddenly I felt something in my jaw shift. She did not apply enough pressure to adjust my jaw physically—it just happened. I'm not sure how. The same happened with my neck. The session lasted an hour and a half. The benefits were amazing.

My jaw, neck, and back pain diminished greatly. I started seeing her twice a week. I stopped suffering those injections into my jaw, ears, neck, and back. The cranial sacral work was far more helpful—and physically painless. It was more than just a physical treatment, though.

The woman would talk to me as well. I would close my eyes and she would ask me "where I was." Almost every time, I would be thinking about the accident. She would talk me through it:

"Where do you see yourself?"

"I'm in the car..." I would tense up, frightened, reliving the accident.

"What do you see?"

"I see that white light again..."

And then I would sob and sob and sob. Reliving the trauma of the accident and the experience of seeing that white light were incredibly powerful and emotional experiences. She took me back there each session and it was terrible. What I realized, of course, was that I had not gotten over the trauma and fear of the accident. It was still inside me. By reliving that trauma with this calm, healing, empathic woman, I was able to somehow slowly release it. Trauma like this can fester. Without letting it out, it only grows.

The cranial sacral work sessions were very intense, emotionally. Still they were noninvasive, gentle, and greatly beneficial. I would leave there feeling as if I had just had the best massage, relieved of any stress, completely relaxed, with no anxiety.

So again I made progress while Mom was visiting, and again she realized there came a point when I was feeling better and she was as much getting in my hair as helping out. After about two weeks Mom went home again after this, her third trip.

My friend Lauryn, who had lost her mother to depression-related suicide, had been trying to get me out of the house. Lauryn was a true friend. At that time she worked as a bartender at Delicious, a fine-dining restaurant and one of my favorite places. The bar inside Delicious had a *Cheers*-type atmosphere where regulars would sit around, socializing. Lauryn was really the heart and soul of the place and created that environment.

For weeks Lauryn had been inviting me to come into the restaurant. Most of the times I made some excuse not to go. A few times I agreed but then I wouldn't make it. I had the best intentions, but showering and getting dressed left me completely fatigued. I would get myself all set to go—and then need to lie back in bed, exhausted. It only made me more depressed. I couldn't even do something as simple as literally getting myself dressed and out of the house.

A few days after Mom left, Lauryn tried again. She put our friend, Andre, on the phone. Andre Reed was a retired NFL player and dear friend. He pushed, in a nice way, to get me to say I'd come out. He was very charming and supportive, joking, telling me we'd have a nice time. He was also very understanding of my situation. Junior Seau, the NFL player who had recently committed suicide, had been Andre's good friend. Andre told me to just come in, have a glass of water, and sit with him. Reluctantly, I finally agreed.

I showered, got dressed, and every little bit of me just wanted to climb back into bed. I had spent all my energy. But then Jordan started encouraging me to go.

"Just say hi, Mom. Even if it's for a minute. Go, Mom, get out of the house."

So I did it. But when I walked into the bar area of the restaurant, I was overwhelmed with how many people were in there. It felt confusing and frustrating simply to see so many people crowded in one place. The voices, the lights, the laughter, the people pushing past me, the clinking of the glasses—it was an assault on my senses, complete overstimulation. I stood in the entranceway to the bar and thought about turning right around when Andre saw me. He walked over with a drink of water. Andre didn't push. He was extremely gentle and understanding. He told me it was okay if I just wanted to chill out and stand there by myself for now, outside the main bar. So that's what I did. After a while the bar started emptying out and I went to sit down with Andre and Lauryn.

We started chatting and immediately I started having problems. I couldn't articulate. I would be in mid-sentence and I'd simply forget what I was about to say. Then I'd get stuck on a word, not be able to find it, and I'd stutter. It was horrifying. I had always been well spoken and expressive. Now I was, again, brain-injury girl. I'd tell them sorry, that I forgot what I was saying or that it wasn't really important—but it didn't matter. Lauryn and Andre were true friends. They knew what had happened to me. They were patient and understanding. There was no judgment, only support. In all it was an embarrassing and exhausting experience. And I couldn't thank them enough for it. I couldn't think of two more special friends to have at my side.

After that Jordan and I had a few date nights but they didn't end well. I used to take my sweet time at restaurants. I loved people watching. I wanted to stay and enjoy the atmosphere. Jordan would always be the one to push me out of the restaurant. Nowadays, though, whenever someone walked by our table it affected me. Somehow they were imposing on my space, my senses. It made me very anxious. Even when a restaurant wasn't loud or crowded—it still felt loud and crowded. We would eat and run. I just couldn't stay inside a public place in those days.

I tried to live my life as normally as possible. On the good days I'd go to the grocery store, run errands—really, I was barely doing anything in terms of what used to be "normal." But like Mom had told me, I had a new normal. This new normal meant that almost every good day was followed by three bad days of sleeping around the clock, feeling mentally and physically fatigued, and emotionally volatile.

I knew Mom was right but—nothing about my life felt normal in any way, shape, or form. At least, it didn't feel like this was a "normal" that I would be able to live with indefinitely. It felt dreadful. There was so much random up and down, back and forth in those days. It was extremely frustrating. I didn't understand the patterns. I'd have positive thoughts one day, see improvement, and then I'd be back in bed, hopeless, for three.

Some days were worse than others. Some were off-the-charts terrible. One day in mid-May stands out.

The words "mental anguish" are easy to write but difficult to really explain. I never knew that one could feel so much pain, mentally. It was an overwhelming combination of pressure and complete misery. Physically my head would feel like it was going to cave in under its own weight, like it was in a vise. Mentally, it felt like there was no hope at all: all there was, all *I* was, was pain.

It had been nearly four months of agony. Some days I didn't know if it was the pain I was feeling that day that was making me completely despondent, or the memory of the pain I had been feeling for the past four months, or the thought that this would be how I lived every day until I died… But whatever it was, on days like these, it was just too much. I felt like I was living in a mental torture chamber. Everything hurt. I wished that I had had every single bone in my body broken rather than feel what I was feeling.

Jordan came home from school on this day in mid-May, walked into my room, and I was lying on my bed, crying hysterically, with both of my hands full of pills.

I don't know what they were, some pain medication they had given me months earlier. I didn't care. All I knew at that minute was I needed the pain to stop.

I can't, I can't, I can't do this anymore. It hurts too much!

"Mom?"

I cried all the harder. How could I let my son see me like this?

Jordan sat down next to me. "Mom, c'mon. Don't be stupid."

Jordan saved my life that day. I didn't know what else to do. I was not in my right mind. But if Jordan hadn't walked in at that exact moment, I absolutely would have swallowed every single one of those pills.

Financially I was still drowning. Clients still dropped off groceries or meals at my door, and it was a blessing. I had borrowed from friends and family, Mom had helped out where she could, but I knew I needed to make some money. Darrah came up with a proactive plan in mid-June. I did not feel able to deal with the overstimulation of the salon, so she suggested I contact my clients and see if they'd come to my place to have their hair done. My clients were sweethearts. Everyone I asked said yes. I was grateful to have a little money coming in.

Jordan's graduation was finally near. It was the one thing I had told myself I wanted to be here for. After that, I secretly didn't care what happened to me.

Four or five days before graduation, Mom came out. My brothers visited as well. We all went out to dinner the night before Jordan's graduation.

I was looking forward to Jordan's graduation. Financially it was going to be a severe challenge, but I was excited by his plans to go to college in Santa Barbara—until they sprang quite a surprise on me at dinner that night.

Jordan had been talking to my mom and my brothers behind my back. He didn't plan on going to college at all.

Jordan's new plan was to become a firefighter. And it wasn't even exactly "new." Shortly after our car accident, Jordan told me at dinner, firefighters came to his high school for career day. One of them had been mentoring Jordan ever since. Jordan had been visiting the fire station and the academy, he had even taken an EMT course—and I had known nothing about it.

Jordan was apologetic at dinner. He didn't want to stress me out, he said, so he hadn't told me.

The first thing out of my mouth was, "Well why don't you tell me what I need to know, not what you think I want to hear—because *that* stresses me out!"

We had driven up to Santa Barbara to look at places for him to live. He had gone up to take his entrance exams. He had told me was going to try out for the football team… I had been spending time and energy planning college with him when I could barely take care of myself. And all the while he had been talking to my mom and brothers about not going—and lying to me.

The truth was, it made sense. The way Jordan had taken control of our car accident scene had been amazing. He was a teenager and yet he was totally calm and collected. Me, I would have run away as fast and far as possible. Jordan had a gift. It wasn't the fact that Jordan had been making plans to be a firefighter that bothered me. It was the fact that he had kept it from me.

We had always communicated so well. We were each other's best friend. Now he had seen me throttle him, scream at him, swear at God, kick him out of the house, and nearly commit suicide on two different occasions. There was no way he could truly understand where I was at. I knew that.

At dinner, after thinking about it, I told Jordan it was his life and his decision. I would support him whatever he chose to do.

Jordan was relieved. My mom and brothers too. But it was very depressing for me.

My family rallied for Jordan's graduation. It was a beautiful ceremony and we had a great party afterward. I couldn't have been more grateful to see him graduate and be surrounded by my family and good friends. After everything I had been through, it was a day of bliss. One thought, though, kept nagging at me.

Jordan had lied to me for months about college. He couldn't count on me like he used to. Were we really best friends? How could we be? I wasn't there for him like before. He couldn't tell me things. The sad truth was, I was unable to be the mom I had always been. It was all because of my injury. It was one more thing that car accident had taken from me—my relationship with my son.

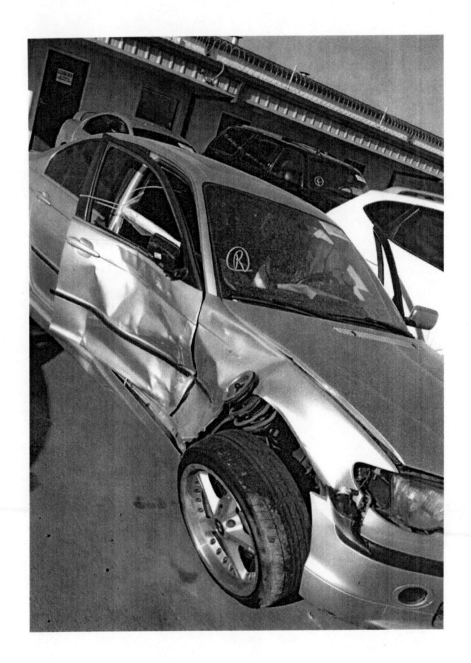

The BMW that saved my life.

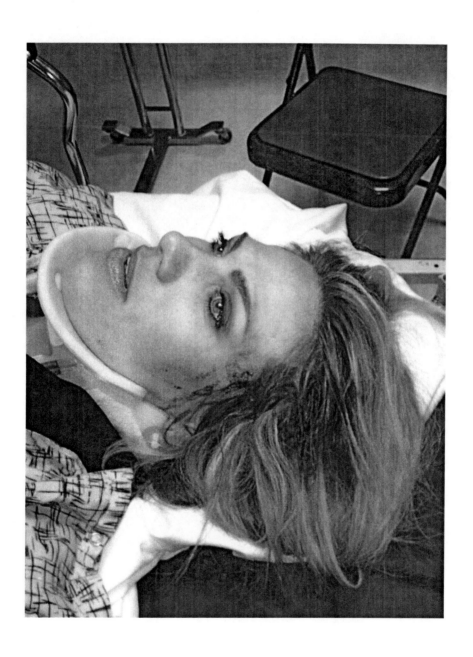

ER Trauma....Scripps La Jolla

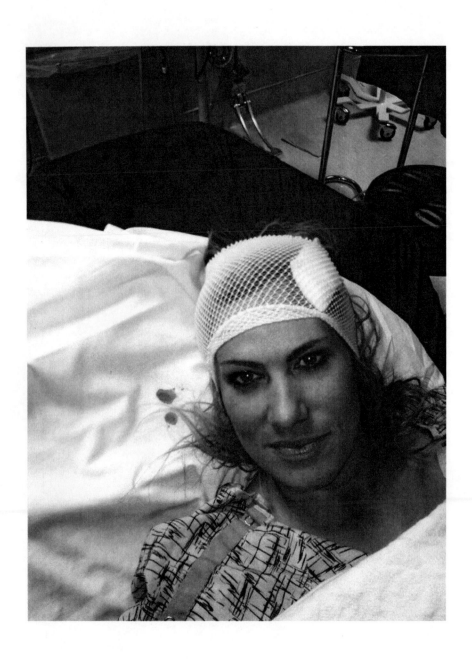

In the Hospital Scripps La Jolla

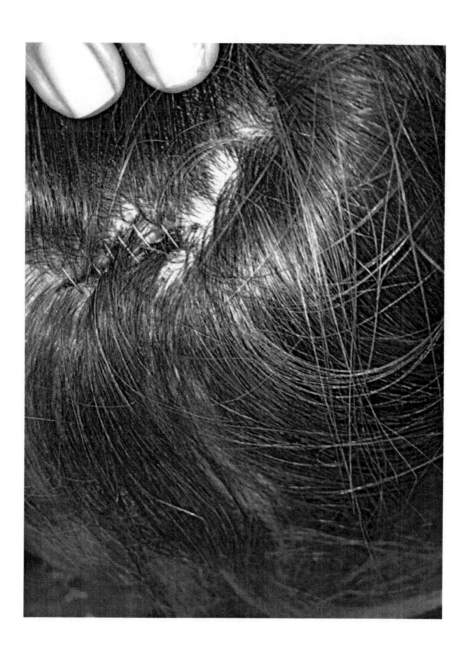

Stapled up

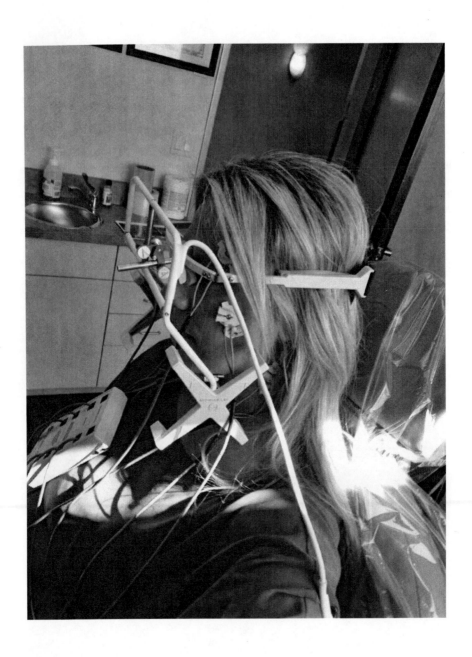

Testing at Scripps La Jolla

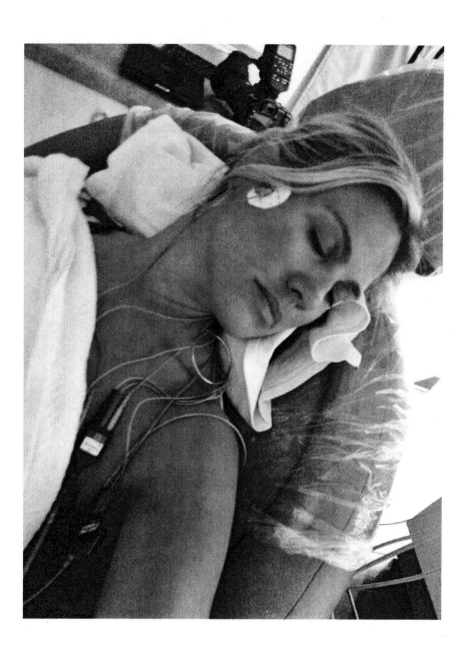

EEG testing

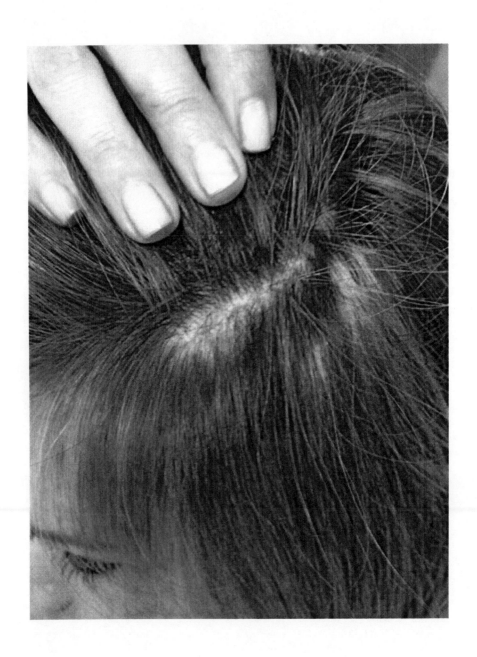

Staples out!!

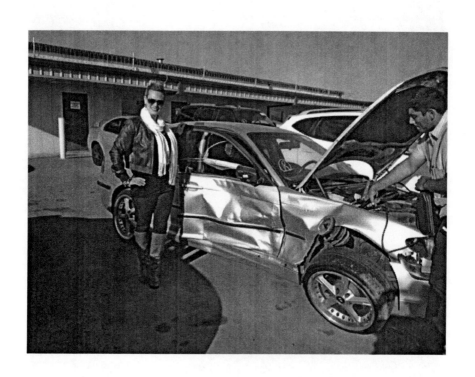

Reunited with the car (BMW) that saved my life.

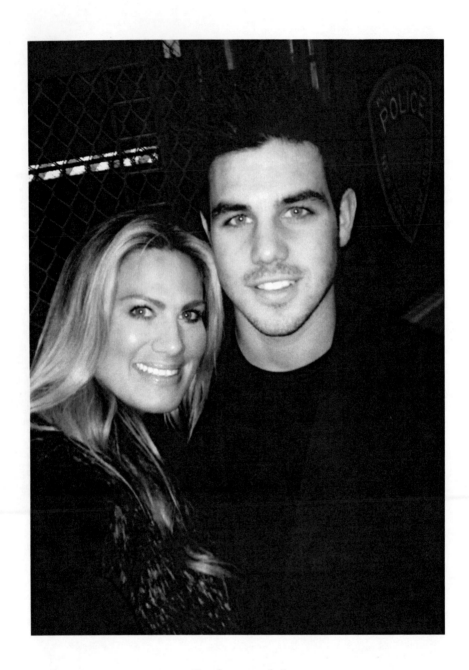

Jordan and I

CHAPTER 7

THE FOLLOWING YEAR –
MORE UPS, MORE DOWNS

July 2012 – June 2013

A month after Jordan's graduation, I moved into a tiny studio apartment in La Jolla. Moving was a serious burden, physically and mentally, but I couldn't afford to stay in the condo I had been living in with Jordan. It was sad because I loved that place and had been there for five years. Jordan started renting a room in Darrah's house.

I had read that isolation was very bad for people who had suffered brain injuries, or for people who suffered from depression. Being alone so much could amplify other issues—fear of leaving the house, anxiety of being around other people, etc. But financially, I didn't have a choice.

Lauryn and Andre successfully got me out of the house a few more times. It was nice to have that support and encouragement. Showering, dressing, and driving somewhere were still exhausting, but I knew it was good for me to get out.

The weeks passed. Clients came to my house so I had a little money coming in. Though all of my symptoms were still there, they were more manageable. That had a lot to do with the antidepressants I was taking. But overall I was feeling better than the previous months.

In August, Darrah convinced me to accompany her on a work

trip to Chicago. We went for a long weekend. In Chicago I happened to meet a guy who was producing an Internet show in Miami. We struck up a conversation, got along, he told me I'd be perfect to host his Internet show, and, just like that, he offered me the job. It was a "meant to be" situation.

I flew back to California and grabbed a few quick sessions with my hosting coach in Los Angeles. I was nervous. Would I be articulate enough to be on camera? Would I freeze up, stutter, forget what I was saying, get stuck mid-sentence, and basically do a million other horrible things that would betray me as brain-injury girl?

Three weeks later I was in Miami, on camera. I hosted an on-location talk show and an inside sports-type show called Press Pass. I was interviewing various personalities and sports celebrities in Miami, including press conference interviews with NFL coaches and players. I knew I wasn't really on my game as far as hosting went. But it wasn't a disaster either. It gave me a little confidence. I realized that I could do this again. I could get back on camera.

For the next few months I would spend eight days in Miami, then ten days back in San Diego. Traveling back and forth was very tiring. I would drag myself home from the airport, crawl into bed, and sleep for a day. Mom was worried that flying was not good for people who had suffered brain injuries, and truly I got fatigued very quickly after what used to be the simplest of activities. But I was determined to regain some sense of continuity with what my life had been like before the accident. It truly was a gift to be back doing what I loved the most, and to have a renewed sense of purpose.

There were good days and bad days, but I was trying to listen to my body. When I needed rest, I rested. Or at least, most of the time. I was learning to be more in tune with my body. And the meds helped. There was definitely some frustration because I still wasn't functioning, mentally, up to my old par. There was still physical pain. I still felt the emotional and mental anguish at times. But things were generally better than they had been the previous months. I figured it was the combination of being busy, being happy to be on camera, the antidepressants, and time simply passing. I felt like I was healing.

While in San Diego, off and on during those months, I spent more and more time at Darrah's house, hanging out with Darrah and Jordan. At one point in November I gave up the La Jolla studio apartment and moved into Darrah's. It made sense and Darrah was all for it. For me, being around Darrah and Jordan was definitely better than being by myself.

I finished working on the Miami show in January 2013. I was able, now, to get around a lot better on my own, so I started driving to my clients' houses to do their hair.

As the first few months of 2013 passed I still didn't have the energy to socialize the way I had in the past, and that was discouraging. I noticed another change in my personality as well. I became impulsive. I lost a dear friend of mine in Los Angeles because I had a conversation with him where I was very abrupt and, frankly, I said harsh, hurtful things. He didn't understand that this was yet another symptom of my brain injury or PCS. At the time, I didn't even realize it. He thought I was just being mean. The truth is—he was right. I had been mean. And it upset me greatly. This just wasn't me. He was the first friend I had made in L.A., many years ago, and I lost him.

I also started drinking impulsively. In fact, following a friend from the Beverly Wilshire in Los Angeles back to his home, I got pulled over and charged with a DUI. The valet had changed my headlight settings so my lights were out. That's what I was pulled over for. But of course that's no excuse. No one should drink and drive, ever. It's something I never would have done in the past. I was always anti–drinking and driving and had lectured Jordan about it all the time.

Again, it was impulsive behavior that just wasn't me.

I grew more and more tired of explaining myself and my behavior. How do you explain to someone that you just drank too much, or you were rude to them, because your personality had shifted due to the brain trauma you had suffered in a car accident? Even to my own ears it sounded like an excuse.

One of the most frustrating parts about the whole thing was: the damage was on the inside. I looked fine. But I often felt crazy. I wanted to move on from it, stop talking about it. I wanted to cover it up, even with my own family. I was tired of discussing how depressed I felt, how sad it all was. Which only made me feel more isolated.

Of course, the insurance company covering the guy who'd crashed into Jordan and me demanded that I see their doctors. If we went to trial, it would be their doctors against mine, fighting over how severe my brain injury was. My own doctors had a "wait and see" plan. I often felt like they discounted much of what I told them. That was incredibly frustrating. But now I had to go to appointment after appointment with doctors whose jobs were, by definition, to *really* discount what I was going through. It wasn't like they were trying to help me. The last thing they wanted to do was order further treatment. Of course they were pleasant, and I understood the nature of the insurance game, but these doctors' purpose was to *not* find anything wrong with me. And there were *many* of them.

The process was extremely time-consuming and fatiguing. Dragging myself to all these appointments was exhausting. And for what? For them to *not* try and help me but instead gather ammunition against me. This is how I spent the first half of 2013, after my Miami hosting jobs finished—trying my best to do as many hair appointments as I could, at home or at my clients' houses, and keeping up with a jam-packed schedule of appointments with the insurance company's doctors. Going to my own doctors was a terrible chore. Going to all these appointments with "opposing" doctors was much, much worse. It felt like all I was doing was talking about my pain. It was like a full-time job.

In June 2013, one of my hair clients went out of town and

invited me to stay at their home. It was just Jordan, our dog, Sammy, and me. The house was on a golf course. The sun was shining, the breeze was blowing. We were lying out by the pool. Everything was beautiful. In all, it was the most carefree, stress-free environment you could imagine. And lying there by the pool, I just started crying. And crying. Uncontrollably.

Jordan asked me what was wrong.

Sobbing, all I could say was, "It's happening again."

Jordan knew what I was talking about. "Mom, look where you are. Look around you. What could be so bad?"

But it didn't matter how happy the situation was, or should have been.

The mental anguish came rushing back. I could literally feel it coming on. Terrible, negative thoughts were barging their way into my brain, pushing every other thought out: it hurt too much. I would be better off gone. I can't do this anymore. And I'm a burden. It'd be better for everyone else if I weren't here. They'd all be better off without me.

I cried and cried. It was like sitting in the car outside Bikram. It was like sitting on my bed with fistfuls of pills when Jordan had walked in on me.

My life was great. There was no stress. Even financially there was no imminent danger. So why was I crying hysterically, thinking that everyone would be better off without me? What was triggering this? Why was it still happening, sixteen months after my accident?

Again, thank God for Darrah. I called her and she was there for me.

"Hannah, you need to shut off your brain," she said. "Take something to knock yourself out and go to bed. Turn those thoughts off. Sleep through this."

She was right so that's what I did. But this time, I was going to hold myself accountable. I would call my doctor and let him know that, even now, long after a year had passed, I still was not mentally and physically okay. We had waited the year. That milestone was behind me and I was still suffering the symptoms. I had been my own advocate with my doctors, I had done my own research, but now something had to change. And it had to come from me.

CHAPTER 8

A GLIMPSE OF LIGHT

July – October 2013

I told myself I was going to get myself healthy. I had to be more pro-active. I have always had a healthy diet, but now I took it more serious-ly. I researched foods that were good for the brain. I started downing fish oil, blueberries, avocadoes—everything specialists said was good for the brain. I had a serious craving for eggs and ate loads of them.

Several months earlier I had taken myself off Zoloft, the antide-pressant. Though my doctor had started me on 10 mg per day back in April of 2012, he had slowly ramped up the dosage. I had been up to 150 mg per day. Though the Zoloft had helped me function, it had also numbed me. I had been walking around flat-lined, dead to the world. I hated that feeling. But now, after my third incident of hav-ing serious thoughts of suicide, I decided to go back on it. It wasn't an easy choice but it seemed to be for the best. Then I read that one side-effect of Zoloft was "suicidal thoughts." You gotta be kidding me, I thought. How wonderful for people who were already depressed. I was damned if I did and damned if I didn't.

I had been seeing my neurologist every six weeks since the acci-dent. He had resisted sending me for a PET scan as well as sending me to other specialists. Now, though, at my insistence, he finally sent me to a neuropsychologist for testing.

I had several sessions with her that lasted two or three hours each. The mental strain to focus on the questions she asked me was exhausting. Afterward, I would drag myself home, climb into my bed, and I wouldn't leave it for three days. I would be completely mentally exhausted. It felt like I had two bodies: my physical body and my mental body. My physical body could go running for hours. But mentally, everything shut down.

During my sessions with the neuropsychologist, she noticed that I would sometimes stare into space for a while, off in my own world. Other times I would forget what she had just asked me. One time I fell asleep sitting at her table with my head in my hands. She said it was possible I was having petit mal seizures. This would account for the blackouts and incidents of falling asleep. She ordered an EEG.

I had been asking my neurologist for a PET scan since day one, and now they wanted to test me for seizures? It's hard to diagnose brain injuries, I knew that. A doctor can't look at you and see what's damaged in your brain, the way he can look at you and see that your arm is broken. With the PET scan, we could possibly see the exact nature of the brain damage, the parts of the brain that were affected, and decide on a course of therapy. I asked my neurologist about it again and he said that if I was showing signs of seizure, we needed to rule that out first.

The EEG test meant that for three and a half days I had to be hooked up to a machine at home, housebound. There was a skullcap with wires—I looked like Frankenstein's monster, a freak of nature. I couldn't leave the house.

The EEG came back clear.

I saw my neurologist shortly after. I was very frustrated. He had always told me he would keep me under observation for a year and see what happens. It had been a year and a half since the accident. This doctor saw me once every six weeks for ten minutes. I was pretty sure I knew my body better than he did. Something was still very wrong and without the proper information, I didn't know how to heal myself.

I dragged myself to his office. This time, though, I didn't dress well or fix myself up like all the previous visits. It had been Darrah's idea. Let him see me as I really was.

Well, it wasn't pretty. I barely had the energy to get myself there. No makeup, no pretty dress; I showed up looking the way I did at home. One of the problems with this kind of injury is when you look good on the outside, everybody just says, "What's wrong with you? You look fine."

I was lying on the table when he entered the exam room. I wasn't going to put on a brave face this time. I told him I was sorry but I didn't have the energy to get up. It was true.

My neurologist sat down, looked at me, put his hand on my knee, and said, "Hannah. You're going to be okay. I think you've had some situational depression. There's a lot going on in your life..." He was so condescending I nearly went through the roof.

I interrupted him, practically shouting. "Are you kidding me?! Do you think I'm sitting here in your office because it's fun?!"

I laid into him. I was entirely done with feeling like he was discounting what I was telling him. "I had suicidal thoughts last week. Again. What is wrong with me? I... want... the PET scan!"

Without a word he got up and started typing into his laptop. "Okay. I'll get you the PET scan."

My attorney and I knew I should have had a PET scan a long time ago. We had been waiting for my doctor to captain the ship. But he hadn't done it until I flipped out on him.

At least it was finally ordered. It felt like, at last, I had been successful being my own advocate in that regard. It should have happened months earlier. It should have happened a year and a half earlier.

My attorney found a doctor in Los Angeles who would do the PET scan on a lien. I got myself up there as quickly as I could.

The PET scan was intense. They need your brain to be natural and normal so they put you in a quiet room to calm you first. Then they put you into this huge, scary, cold metal tube—and ask you to keep your brain calm and normal.

After the scan, the main doctor came into my room and said they had seen where my injury was. He asked me to go upstairs with him.

Upstairs, he led me into a big conference room. There was a group of doctors sitting around a big table, and huge video screens everywhere with pictures of my brain up on them. I felt immediately like these doctors cared about me.

The main doctor pointed out a spot on the left side of my brain. Most of my brain was showing up very dark, nearly black, with maybe a tiny bit of color here and there. And there, where he pointed, was a white dot. It was like a bruise. It wasn't some big mass, just a white dot.

He told me that that spot was the injury itself, but I was showing signs and symptoms of having injured the right side of my brain also, as well as the frontal lobe... the other doctors were nodding, seriously but compassionately... the main doctor kept talking but in my mind, I was rejoicing. Sure it was scary. They were pointing out this dead spot in my brain and talking about other potentially damaged areas but—I finally had an advocate. I finally felt like I had doctors on my side. And it never would have happened if I hadn't wigged out and screamed at my doctor.

They told me they thought I should have a functional MRI done. It was a more complete scan. The PET scan shows where you have an injury. The functional MRI would show which parts of the brain that injury was affecting. It was very expensive so I called my attorney. He said yes, do it.

They gave me a two-hour break. Then they did the functional MRI.

It was even more intense than the PET scan and very scary. They strapped me down on a stretcher. My torso, arms, legs—everything was velcroed down. They connected a chin guard to my face, then attached one of those halos to my head to keep it still. I couldn't move a muscle. As they slid me into the cold metal tube, I started crying. I felt so alone. There wasn't a big support system for me. I had Mom and Jordan and Darrah—and God bless them—but there was so much I had to go through by myself. I didn't know what I was getting into that day. I thought it'd be a little PET scan, then I'd drive home. I had no idea how physically intense and emotionally draining it would be. No one should have to go through all of this alone.

I was in that tube for forty-five minutes. It was cold. Loud engines were churning all around me. The fact that I was getting these scans done was incredibly encouraging and satisfying. The reality of being up in L.A. alone, though, stuck in this medical complex from eight a.m. till nine p.m., was very difficult.

Still, I felt like I got more done for myself in that one day than I had in the previous year and a half.

My neurologist saw the results of both scans about a week later. He agreed—they showed where the injury was, the impact. They also showed that my brain activity had been affected on the right side, and in the frontal lobe. My neurologist jumped onboard. He told my attorney he'd want to get us his full report before we went to trial.

The location of the areas affected in my brain explained why I was crying all the time, why my mood had been so strongly affected, why I had been so emotionally volatile—they proved what I knew had been going on.

My doctor had told me to give it a year and see where I was at. That year had come and gone and I still wasn't better. My requests for the PET scan hadn't been taken seriously. I was still on medication, still having these symptoms, and I knew my body wasn't right. It was very frightening. Seeing the injury in the PET scan, knowing that the areas affected in my brain showed up in the functional MRI—it gave me some peace. I wasn't crazy. Well, okay, so I kind of was. But at least I knew why and where I was crazy! In a strange way it was comforting to see it all, to see the damaged and affected parts of my brain, physically.

I wished I had had it done much earlier. I might have known better how to rehabilitate myself. It had been such a long time of not knowing. I had been proactive in terms of the cranial sacral work and my diet. I had always been my own advocate but I wished I had spoken out louder, sooner. The more you're educated on the specifics of what's happening, the better you can treat yourself. At least now I knew what was going on. And so did my doctors.

Having the tests done was a major victory, but the war was far from over.

Not long after, I had a fourth incident of considering suicide. I was at home. Nothing unusual was going on, nothing stressful. But I felt those dark thoughts coming on again. Like the previous time, I felt them creeping into my brain, pushing out every other thought: I'm a burden to everyone I love. It would just be better for everyone if I were gone.

This time, though, even as it was happening, I knew what I had to do. It was almost like there were two Hannahs: the one who was feeling these dark thoughts, and the other one, looking on objectively, who knew what she had to do. I thought back to being in that conference room in L.A., looking at the scans of my brain. There's a physical explanation for this, I thought. There's a little white spot of damage on my brain. I pictured it. There are other parts of my brain that, physically, showed up as being affected. It wasn't nebulous, mysterious, unknown—it was fact and I had seen it.

I held myself accountable. The one who was going to have to help me—was me. I took a Xanax and put myself to bed. I was out for twelve hours. The next day, though I had close to zero energy, I felt a little better. I snapped out of it. The last time I had felt suicidal, it had taken three days until I felt more like myself again. This time it was the next day.

The next few months—July, August, and September—were filled

with more visits with the insurance company's doctors. Still it was like a full-time job—appointment after appointment, test after test. It was a miserable way to spend my time. It was like I was living for these appointments with doctors whose very last thought was doing anything to help me or provide me with answers. I didn't have the time to visit friends or take more hosting classes in L.A. My focus had to be these doctor appointments, and it was depressing. I had gained a lot of weight from the medications, which didn't exactly help me feel better about myself.

I weaned myself off the antidepressants. I started skipping a day. Then I skipped two days between pills. I got to the point where I was taking one pill every three days, then one time I simply forgot to take it on the third day. I realized it on the fourth day and said to myself, well, let's just see what happens if I don't take it today either. The next day, I said the same thing to myself. Things went okay and in this way, sort of by mistake, I stopped taking them.

It was a blessing to feel life again. I had much more mental clarity. I was now, more than ever, bound and determined to heal myself. I'd still get angry at Jordan from time to time, but I wouldn't rage. I'd still cry, but it wouldn't cripple me in bed for days and days. Feeling is normal. We're not meant to walk around in a fog, numb, all the time.

My trial date was approaching, November 20. I was completely and utterly sick of the whole thing. We had a mediation and they offered us a very small amount. My doctors were telling me that I could go to trial and be awarded seven million dollars—or nothing. I looked great, they told me. I was pretty and by all appearances I had my act together. I had done my hosting jobs in Miami and the opposing insurance company was using that against me: look, she's flying around the country having a great time, how bad off could she be? The truth was, the hosting job was exactly that—my job. Traveling had been exhausting, filming had been exhausting, but it had brought in money I desperately needed. It was work. I didn't exactly do it for kicks, but their angle was that I was having the time of my life and—look at these videos—she's smiling, laughing, she's obviously healthy.

She looks great.

Well, that's because my disability was invisible.

But it didn't matter to them. It was very, very frustrating.

I waffled back and forth. One day I wanted to go to trial, the next day I just wanted it over. Finally, in late September, I told my attorney to settle the case. I didn't want it hanging over my head during the holidays. I wanted to wipe my hands clean. I wanted it behind me.

In the end, after the doctors and lawyer got their fair share, what I received was very, very little, relatively speaking. But that was okay. I needed to move on with my life.

One day in October I hiked Torrey Pines. I climbed to the top of that rock—the same one I had hiked up back before the accident happened, when I had felt on top of the world, like nothing could stop me.

I sat on the rock, praying. I was thanking God. I was mending. I felt like working out again, exercising. And I was extremely grateful.

A guy came up to me and we started talking. He was a firefighter. He knew the paramedics who had come to our accident scene. He told me that, on the job, he also had suffered brain trauma.

"The doctors had told me to wait a year but that year came and went without much change," he said.

I shook my head. It had been the same for me.

"It took about a year and a half for me to start feeling better," he said.

Hearing that was amazing. Again, it had been pretty much the same for me.

"It'll get better," he said. "You'll start feeling better and better, you'll be able to work out again. Pretty soon you'll be back in the swing of things. It won't be the same," he said, "but you'll be back in a daily routine." It was incredible. This guy was nailing it right on the head. We said our good-byes. I sat on the rock, a bit stunned by the coincidence of running into this guy.

It was like an angel had come to sit with me at Torrey Pines and tell me exactly what I had needed to hear!

I thought back on the other "angels" who had passed through my life in the previous twenty or so months. Brenda, the woman at the car accident who had been so compassionate. My mom, Jordan, Darrah. Andre and Lauryn. Tom Shadyac on the *Ellen* show.

I sat on that rock, overlooking the Torrey Pines gold course and the ocean, and I thought, things will never be the same. Mom was right. I had a "new normal." Bad days still happened, unexplainable moods, crying, mental pain… It had been an extremely hard road, and it wasn't over. But I had been giving a lot of thought recently to what had happened to me and why. My road to recovery had been agonizing and very lonely. I knew there were many, many people out there who'd suffered similar trauma to mine. The brain injury, the PCS, depression, the struggles with the doctors…

I thought about Tom Shadyac and how his brain injury and PCS had changed his life, how he was now a force for so much good through his documentaries and charities. I needed to practice what I preached.

I decided to write a book.

It gave me a new purpose. I would take what had happened to me and reach out to others. I wouldn't pull any punches. I wouldn't paint the picture that it's easy to get past brain injury and PCS. I wouldn't claim that "I've been through it and here's how I got back to the person I was before the injury." That was just not going to happen.

There's a new normal. But I have been given the grace to accept who I am, today.

I would share the idea that every day is a challenge. Every day is a choice. No one is alone. I would encourage people in similar circumstances to be their own advocates where doctors are concerned, to speak up loudly and forcefully. I would do what I could to help create a sense of community amongst those of us who have had these life-changing injuries.

It might not seem like it during the darkest times but—there is hope. Working out, eating right, being healthy—they help. But feeling like you're not alone, finding people like Tom Shadyac and the fire-fighter I had just met—these were truly the biggest helps. None of us are alone.

I decided to share and give back. I would do my best to be an angel for others, the way these people in my life had been angels for me. I would do what I could for those, like me, who had been suffering with their invisible disability.

I would write a book.

If I could help one person, all the pain and anguish I had suffered would be worth it.

I exhibited nearly every one of the above warning signs for suicide. And of course, I came very close to attempting suicide several times.

I took antidepressants for months after I was diagnosed with depression. As I wrote in Part 1, they got me on my feet again; it was like a fog lifted before my eyes. For me, though, being on them was also numbing. I felt like I was walking around flat-lined. I made the mistake of quitting them cold turkey, and I believe that contributed to my next bout with thoughts of suicide. Plus, one of the potential side-effects of my antidepressant was "may have suicidal thoughts." Crazy right?

Again, every case is different and I am not a doctor. But people suffering from PCS and/or depression need to educate themselves. Ask your doctor. Try not to be ashamed of investigating the possibility that you may be suffering from depression. Be your own advocate, hold yourself accountable, and take responsibility for your own recovery. It's not easy. Ask for help.

I was able to wean myself off antidepressants about a year and a half after my accident. I strongly recommend this weaning method rather than cold turkey, and it's something you need to discuss with your doctor. But the bottom line is: educate yourself, talk openly with your doctor, and if your doctor doesn't seem to be on the same page as you—push the issue. Seek a second opinion.

PART 3

Healing from the Inside Out

Below are ten tips I would like to share, ones that worked for me during my recovery. During the first part of my journey recovering from PCS and depression, I was not able to fully appreciate and process them. Now, two years after my car accident, these basically represent the best advice I can give.

Again, I am not a doctor. I'm a pragmatist. I believe the below are valuable for people dealing with PCS and depression, as well as for their caregivers.

10 Tips to Healing Yourself from the Inside Out

1 – ACCEPTANCE

- Give yourself the grace to accept who you are today rather than who you used to be yesterday.
- There's a "new normal."
- There will be times when it's "one step forward and two steps back." It will be extremely frustrating.
- Take one day at a time. In fact, take life moment by moment.
- Things will never get better until you accept your injury and who you are now.

2 – LISTEN TO YOUR BODY

- You have the power to heal yourself. Your body is a natural healing vehicle. You are the divine healer within. Your body knows exactly what to do to heal itself. Listen to it.
- You are the physician of your own mental, physical, and

spiritual well-being.

- If your body is telling you that you are tired—sleep. If you feel overstimulated at home, put yourself in a quiet, dark room.
- Be mindful of medications. Their side-effects may be more hazardous to you than the medication is helpful to your symptom. For instance, Zoloft made me crave sugar and bad carbs— breads, pastas—foods that cause depression. Limit yourself on meds if possible. Less is more.

3 – BE YOUR OWN ADVOCATE

- I found that I knew my body at times better than my doctors did.
- Even if you are talking to your doctor and she has a different opinion than you—don't discount what your body is telling you.
- Don't be afraid to show your doctor what's truly going on. I put on a tough, happy face for my doctor, so every time I was in his office I looked fine.
- This disability is invisible; you have to be clear and honest about how you're feeling.
- My doctor wasn't listening to me until I put my foot down. You're paying your doctor. Speak up and be firm.
- Bring notes to your medical appointments. Before my doctor visits, I used to write up a list of questions and symptoms I had been experiencing. The minute you get in there you might forget what you wanted to tell your doctor.
- Keep a journal. Write things down daily, your feelings and symptoms. Bring it with you to your appointments. Even if it's just three words for one day. Believe me, you will forget how you were feeling. It'll help you remember things to tell your doctor. Also, going back and reading it later is eye opening. It will help you understand how far you've come or how far you've regressed.

4 – BRAIN FOODS AND HYDRATION

BRAIN FOODS

I strongly believe that eating "brain foods" sped up my healing process. You will find many lists online of foods that deliver nutrients to as well as flush toxins from the brain. There are loads of scientific studies to read.

On a practical note, I found it helpful to get a juicer. Many people who experience PCS suffer painful jaw problems like TMJ. Others lose their sense of taste. Eating can be painful; it can be a chore. My mom got me a juicer early into my recovery. It was a great idea and helped me get the proper nutrients I probably wouldn't have gotten otherwise.

Below are the foods I feel strongly about, from my own research and experience.

- **Blueberries** – Blueberries are usually at the top of every list of brain foods, for good reason. Blueberries are packed with nutrients that improve brain function, and they are easily absorbed into the bloodstream and processed by the brain. I found myself craving them during my recovery. I would eat a pint in one sitting. I believe my body was telling me what it needed.

- **Other fruits and vegetables** – Studies show that diets high in fruits and vegetables seem to improve cognitive and motor functions, especially dark-colored fruits and veggies such as strawberries, avocados, bananas, tomatoes, and dark greens (kale, spinach, Brussels sprouts, broccoli, etc.).

- **Fish oils** – Fish oils contain high levels of Omega 3 fatty acids. These are great for just about every system in the body. You can make sure to eat lots of fish, but many fish gather contaminants and mercury as they grow, especially larger, older fish.

My advice is to take fish oil as a supplement. I used to take 5000 mg a day.

- **Other foods that deliver EFAs** – Essential Fatty Acids such as Omega 3 – include nuts and seeds, algae, chia seeds, olive oil, and coconut oil.
- **Proteins** – During my recovery, I found myself craving eggs. More specifically, egg yolks. Then I found that egg yolks contain high levels of choline, a nutrient that boosts brainpower by increasing the speed of the signals sent between nerve cells in the brain. Other proteins that contain nutrients and antioxidants beneficial to the brain include dairy products, chicken, lean red meats, liver, cannelloni beans, and goat's milk.
- **Dark chocolate** – Dark chocolate is packed with antioxidants. It releases endorphins, giving us a natural pick-me-up. Dark chocolate also contains high concentrations of theobromine, which is a natural stimulant to help keep us focused without stimulating the central nervous system, like coffee does.
- **Whole grains and brown rice** – Good cereals and breads, oats, rye, quinoa, millet, brown rice—they all are excellent brain foods that improve circulation and deliver folic acids, fibers, and vitamins that are especially helpful in building and flushing the brain.
- If possible, avoid completely:
- **Refined sugars** – Sugar causes brain inflammation, reduces brain cell function, helps other toxins enter the brain more easily, and causes depression anxiety.
- **Complex carbohydrates** – White flour or white bread can actually intensify feelings of depression.
- **Alcohol** – Alcohol intensifies many emotional and cognitive problems, and not just while you're actually drinking.

HYDRATION

Keeping hydrated is extremely important. The first signs of dehydration are headache, malaise, problems focusing, problems with short-term memory, and general mental fogginess. Those of us suffering from PCS or depression have enough going on in these departments without compounding it all with dehydration!

Don't just drink water; drink *good* water. Our brains are 85% water. Given that fact, think about just how important *which* water we drink is.

Tap water may contain contaminants and additives. Many brands of bottled water are really tap water in a bottle and still contain contaminants and chlorine.

My mother introduced me to Kangen Water. I strongly suggest it. You can find out more about it at www.kangenlivingh2o.com.

This website will tell you that Kangen Water's cellular structure is "micro-clustered," much smaller than ordinary tap water, so it can be absorbed into the cells and brain more quickly. Kangen Water includes antioxidants. It is alkaline and ionized water, which means it reduces acidity and dehydration.

For whatever the reason, I responded strongly to Kangen Water.

5 – FAMILY AND COMMUNITY

- Don't isolate yourself. It is extremely important to have the right friends and family members around you. One of the first things a person with PCS will be inclined to do is isolate him- or herself—but isolation will just make things worse.
- All of us with PCS need what I call in-your-face friends— friends who do more than call or text. The friends of mine who truly cared were the ones who showed up at my door with meals, groceries, or gifts of money. Those were the ones who stuck around.

- Learn to put your pride and ego aside and accept help. More than that, learn to ask for it. Being a strong, independent woman, one of the hardest things for me was to receive help let alone ask for it. It's okay for your friends and family to want to help you—including financially. In fact, it's a blessing, especially as many with PCS struggle to hold down a job due to problems focusing and staying on task.

- Even a dog helps! During my recovery, I inherited a puppy, Sammy. Sammy gave me unconditional love. Just to have him next to me in my dark times was very comforting. Sammy also gave me a purpose, a reason to get out of bed sometimes. I found that having a puppy was incredibly healing and gave me a responsibility other than myself that wasn't overwhelming.

For caregivers:

- Be patient.
- Accept the new normal of your loved one.
- Love them for who they are now, not who they were before. Be open to change.
- Remember that mood swings and outbursts are common symptoms. Don't take things personally when they rage.
- Remember that, underneath everything, no one wants to be left alone. The person with the injury won't reach out. You have to physically take action. Go to them.
- My son, Jordan, will tell you: the last thing a caregiver wants to say is, "It's all in your head!"
- Remember that this disability is invisible. It often doesn't look like anything's wrong. Physically, visually—you can't tell.
- Get informed. Read up on signs and symptoms. Google. Educate yourself.
- Help your loved one with PCS break down lists into doable tasks. Help them to not get overwhelmed.

- Be mindful that the simplest tasks can be incredibly hard for someone suffering symptoms of PCS—showering and cooking never mind driving and shopping.

6 – THE POWER OF POSITIVE THINKING AND A GOOD SENSE OF HUMOR

- **Positive thinking** – I cannot stress enough the importance of positive thinking and a positive mindset. Stay positive even in the darkest days. Hang onto one positive mantra and repeat it. In the midst of the worst of it, you won't see anything positive. So visualize yourself as being well at some point in the future—and wait for your body to catch up.
- **Organize your thoughts** – One thing that helped me immensely was creating a vision board. I put together images and words that I wanted for myself in the future. It helped me stay on target and it has been incredibly powerful to see them come to fruition, like—writing this book!
- **Change your mindset** – You can change your way of life by changing your mind.
- **Perspective** – The gift of perspective is the greatest gift in life. The key to life is looking at the glass half full. No matter the situation, you can always walk away with something positive. Stepping into my doctor's office and seeing some of his unfortunate other patients often gave me a good sense of perspective. Someone always has it worse. Appreciate what you have as opposed to focusing on what you don't have.
- **Gratitude** – I get up in the morning thanking God for each day, for what I *do* have. I think about what a great day it's going to be. It puts me on the right foot.
- **Humor** – The importance of laughter and humor is huge. Laugh with yourself, laugh at yourself. For me, at many times, I had to either laugh about things—or cry. It helps those

around you too.

- My girlfriends would joke with me, saying: "Hannah, you always had brain problems, now you just have an excuse!"
- I'd make jokes like: "I know I should be stressing about something but I don't remember what it is. Oh yeah, my rent is due tomorrow. I only have $700 and it's $2,500—oh yeah, I should be stressing about that!"

7 – PROPER EXERCISE

For me, the benefits of Bikram yoga were amazing. It literally healed me from the inside out, cell by cell, head to toe.

Some benefits of Bikram yoga include:

- The poses and the heat help increase blood flow, which means more energy.
- Some positions specifically target increasing blood flow to the brain, which helps bring brain cells "out of cold storage."
- The emphasis on breathing patterns helps focus the mind, improve clarity, and reduce stress.
- Chronic pain is diminished as strength and flexibility improve.
- The heat warms the muscles for greater flexibility, flushes toxins, and improves the immune system. The heat also helps expand the blood vessels, flushing circulation and helping with low blood pressure, sexual vitality, and overall health.
- Overall, Bikram yoga brings balance to the body's systems: skeletal, muscular, circulatory, nervous, digestive, respiratory—you name it.

Bikram worked for me and I recommend it wholeheartedly. Ultimately, though, you need to find what works for *your* body—and do it. Maybe start with something small. Yoga was good for me partially because it was not too strenuous, it was easy on the body—it was doable.

Whatever exercise is good for you, push yourself to do it. Find an accountability partner and exercise with them. Of course consult your doctor first, but exercise gets the endorphins going and that helps to eliminate depression.

I can't stress enough how important exercise truly is for treating depression.

8 – EXPLORE ALTERNATIVE TREATMENTS

There is a time for Western medicine and there is a time for Eastern medicine. I have my mom to thank for much of the research into alternate forms of healing that benefited me. Not everyone has the drive to pursue these things for themselves, especially as they suffer from symptoms of PCS. If you need help investigating alternative forms of treatment, ask for it.

I'm a pragmatist. Scientific proof and the complete understanding of underlying causes are still the gold standard for Western medical practice, but in their absence, my criteria is strictly pragmatic. I go by results. You try one thing. If it doesn't work, you try another. That was my own personal approach.

- **Cranial sacral work** was incredibly helpful for me. I strongly encourage people suffering from PCS to try it.
- **Essential oils** such as Rosemary, Basil, Juniper Berry, Peppermint, and Sage or Clary Sage help increase mental clarity. Some may be ingested under the tongue or worked into the skin; others can be dropped into boiling water or circulated with a candle diffuser.
- **Massages** help too. Listen to your body and get the type of massage you feel like you need—relaxation versus deep tissue, etc. Massage is great for flushing toxins and getting things flowing through your body.

These are alternative treatments that worked for me. Other people have had success with acupuncture and hypobaric chambers. Take this information, do your own research, and find what works for you.

Overall, keep an open mind.

9 – ACCOUNTABILITY

- Be proactive about your own healing. No one's going to do it for you.
- Early on during my journey of recovery, I was unable to be accountable for myself. I would spiral down so far that I just couldn't reach out. For me, it took over a year to truly hold myself responsible for my own healing. Later on in my recovery, though, during my bouts with suicidal thoughts, I held myself accountable by alerting my doctors, family, and closest friend. When those thoughts came, and I recognized them for what they were, it was like—oh my gosh, here we go. I need to tell someone.
- Part of accountability includes watching out for addiction to prescription drugs. In my opinion, less is more. *You* need to keep an eye on yourself.
- Be honest with yourself and your caregivers regarding what your body is telling you. If you're feeling PCS symptoms or suspect you're suffering from depression, tell your loved ones. Tell your doctor. Again—no one is going to do it for you.

10 – FAITH AND PURPOSE

For me, my faith in God was the number one factor that got me through my recovery. It gave me hope in the darkest of days. God will never give you more than you can handle. Beneath every struggle is a reason and thus a purpose. God can take the struggles of today and turn them into the dreams of tomorrow.

Things will get better.

Don't give up.

Redirect your energy into something positive that motivates you in life. Maybe that means giving back to someone else or helping other people.

For me, struggling through PCS and depression, I found myself. I found a purpose: to take my experience and share it, encouraging other people who are suffering from PCS and depression to have hope, to not give up.

Taking your mind off of yourself and directing that energy towards something positive—maybe towards helping other people—will become its own reward.

PART 4

WHERE I'M AT NOW

Living an invisible disability can sometimes be harder than a physical disability. No one can see it, though we live it every moment of the day. Much of the time, we're trying to put on a happy face that says everything inside is just as okay as everything looks on the outside.

At times I wished I had broken every bone in my body so people would see and understand how badly I was hurting.

As I look back on those days, during the worst times of my recovery, the one goal I had was to see Jordan graduate. After that, I thought, I could pass away. But no. I am here today not only living, but thriving and here to talk about it.

I'm not trying to paint a picture that everything is perfect for me because it's not. I have hiccups. Memory loss... short attention span... depression tries to creep in now and then. In those times, I utilize the healing methods I discovered along the way that worked for me—the ones I have described in this book.

It's a lifelong journey.

But I believe it's my choice every day to make it the best day ever. No one, no thing, no disability will keep me down or silenced.

I write this book not for myself, or to be heard, but for those who have suffered from a brain injury, PCS, deep depression, or have a loved one suffering. If it means I help to save one life, then what I went through was worth it, every minute of it.

Writing this book has given me a purpose and passion for others. I plan to write more books. I am developing a talk show, *Hannah Talk*.

My desire is to give people a voice. Everyone has a story and everyone is on his and her own personal journey. No two are the same.

I now have a greater love and empathy for those suffering. I truly believe that as a community, if we raise awareness about PCS and depression, and talk about them rather than minimize them and label or judge those who suffer, we can heal one by one.

No one person should suffer in silence.

You do have a purpose on this planet. Love yourself. You are truly a gift, no matter what anyone says about you—especially those voices in your head. Don't let that chatter in your mind squelch your designed purpose.

You have the power within you to heal yourself. Still, things might be different from here on out. You might have a new normal. But that's okay. Give yourself the grace to accept it—and move forward. Get up every day and put one foot right in front of the other. And know someone loves you to your core.

There is a community, family, and friends who want to support you. Even in your deepest, darkest, most anguished day there is hope. There is always a new day, a new solution, or a new destiny. As God carried me in the palm of His hand the entire journey, I would get glimpses of hope each day. Count your blessings one by one, my friends, even the smallest of the small.

I know, I've been there, and I assure you: there is an end to the pain.

Things will get better.

Never, ever give up.

ACKNOWLEDGEMENTS:

I wish to offer a heartfelt "thank you" from the bottom of my heart: First and foremost to God, the reason I am here today.

To my son & best friend Jordan; I truly have had the honor of raising my best friend. You inspire me in all I do in life, Son. I love you.

To my loving mother (Jo) & stepfather (Vern) with their gentle love and constant support always encouraging me and nurturing my faith.

To my father (Jerry) for all your love.

To my siblings, your love and humor always brings a light into my life: Reneé, David, Stephen & Michael. I love you all.

To my auntie (June Otjen), thank you for always telling me what I needed to hear rather than what I wanted to. I love all our special talks.

To my dear friend Darah and two sons Jack & Beckett; without you three I wouldn't be where I am today. Thank you for showing Jordan and me what true friends really are.

To my big boy (Sammy the dog), thank you for literally always being by my side.

To Dr. Bruce Beutler, you truly have blessed my life in many aspects; thank you for the gift of your knowledge and friendship.

To Andre Reed (HOF), you were that friend always there for me, always there to get me out of the house even when I couldn't.

To Lauryn Evarts, thank you for saving my life and shedding light on the depression I never knew I had. I love you.

To my friend Susanne Schalin, for always dragging me to Bikram; there's no free lunch.

To my ghostwriter Scott Baldyga; you rock in many ways. Thank you for Skyping with me at my worst and bringing my story to a reality.

To all my dedicated family, friends, doctors & nurses, who truly made my recovery a success. You know who you are.

I thank each and every one of you in advance that read this book. I pray a special prayer for you that you may be blessed abundantly in every area of your life.

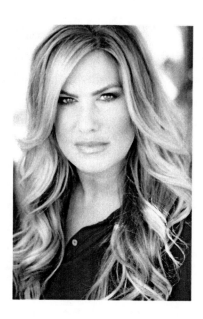

Hannah Andrusky teaches people what it takes to cultivate and exercise resilience. She knows firsthand that life can deal some pretty tough blows. And, for us to not only cope but thrive, we need to have a guide who can offer compassionate and compelling advice.

In 2012 a serious car accident sidelined Hannah's career as talk show host and stylist – as well as her confidence and self-esteem. Her "invisible disability' of concussion syndrome left her depressed, exhausted and even suicidal. Her medications caused her to gain weight and have severe mood swings, contributing to her lack of equilibrium on many fronts. A single mother and a daughter, her caretakers often had had enough of the resulting behaviors.

Hannah, with faith and a keen sense of knowing she experienced these things for a purpose, began acknowledging her struggle publicly, eliciting responses from those with similar issues due to PTSD, illness or the basic trauma of living in our changing world. She chose to become a student of what worked for her in her recovery process, perspective and the perceptions of the gifts she knew she was intended to pay forward. Now, she speaks, teaches, coaches and has authored, Living the Invisible Disability – Healing the Brain from the Inside Out.

Hannah is an advocate for positive and spiritual change, which is the focus of her show, 'Hannah Talk' (www.HannahTalk.com). Noted for her compassionate but candid style (with an edge), Hannah promotes beauty that radiates from the inside out. She believes her accident was a blessing that led her to rediscover her passion for uncovering people's 'real' stories – and helping them see their way through and past them. Through 'Hannah Talks' she helps people find their voice, strength and inner beauty. She leads her clients, participants and viewers to the choice of living life full out, and doing it well.

A successful stylist for 18 years, Hannah worked with clients in Montana, LA, Las Vegas, San Diego, New York and Miami, including celebrities. It was on this 'stage' that she honed her interview style and was encouraged to pursue a media career. She attributes her inspiration to her faith in God, and her son, Jordan. Hannah and Jordan reside in Bel Air, California.

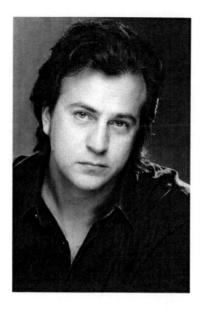

Scott Baldyga is a professional writer and filmmaker. He lives in Los Angeles with his wife and daughter. Scott is thankful to be part of this brave, candid account and believes that raising awareness about PCS and TBI is a much-needed step toward developing a stronger sense of community amongst those who suffer from them. Visit Scott at www.scottbaldyga.com

A Portion of the books proceeds will be dontated to: B.R.A.I.N. Foundation, www.thebrainsite.org & Invisibilities Disabilities Association, www.invisibledisabilities.org

CPSIA information can be obtained at www.ICGtesting.com
Printed in the USA
BVOW01s1717300414

352176BV00001B/238/P